Advancing Health and Well-Being

The Robert Wood Johnson Foundation Culture of Health Series

Series Editor, Alonzo L. Plough

Advancing Health and Well-Being

Using Evidence and Collaboration to Achieve Health Equity

EDITED BY ALONZO L. PLOUGH, PHD, MPH, MA

OXFORD
UNIVERSITY PRESS

OXFORD
UNIVERSITY PRESS

Oxford University Press is a department of the University of Oxford. It furthers
the University's objective of excellence in research, scholarship, and education
by publishing worldwide. Oxford is a registered trade mark of Oxford University
Press in the UK and certain other countries.

Published in the United States of America by Oxford University Press
198 Madison Avenue, New York, NY 10016, United States of America.

Library of Congress Cataloging-in-Publication Data
Names: Sharing Knowledge to Build a Culture of Health Conference (2017 :
Louisville, Ky.), author. | Plough, Alonzo L., editor.
Title: Advancing health and well-being :
using evidence and collaboration to achieve health equity / edited by Alonzo L. Plough.
Other titles: Robert Wood Johnson Foundation culture of health series.
Description: Oxford; New York : Oxford University Press, [2018] |
Series: Robert Wood Johnson Foundation culture of health series |
Includes bibliographical references and index.
Identifiers: LCCN 2018012905 | ISBN 9780190884734 (softcover : alk. paper)
Subjects: | MESH: Health Policy | Health Services | Health Status Disparities |
Economics, Medical | United States | Congresses
Classification: LCC RA418 | NLM WA 540 AA1 | DDC 362.1—dc23
LC record available at https://lccn.loc.gov/2018012905

1 3 5 7 9 8 6 4 2

Printed by Sheridan Books, Inc., United States of America

CONTENTS

SECTION V   PROFILES OF KENTUCKY

FOREWORD

In April 2017, I became the new president and chief executive officer of the Robert Wood Johnson Foundation (RWJF), the nation's largest philanthropy dedicated solely to health. I am honored and energized to lead this organization, and I'm deeply committed to our vision of collaborating with others to build a Culture of Health that benefits all.

Achieving health equity is one of the most important elements of a Culture of Health, so that everyone, in every community, has a fair and just opportunity for health and well-being. This goal resonates with me in a powerful way because I've seen what health *inequity* looks like. As a pediatrician working in a community clinic in New York City, I was struck by the profound difference in opportunities my patients had when compared to children living just a 15-minute subway ride away. I might encourage a family to make healthier choices, like filling their plates with fresh fruits and vegetables or getting the recommended 60 minutes of daily exercise. But the truth is that the choices we make depend on the choices we have available to us. It's heartbreaking to know that the essentials of good health—such as nutritious food, good schools and jobs, and safe places to exercise and play—are out of reach for so many families.

Since 1972, RWJF has aimed to help people achieve the best health possible, no matter where they live or what their physical or economic circumstances might be. We are largely known as a grantmaker, supporting research and programs that target some of the nation's most urgent health issues. As a nonpartisan leader in health philanthropy, RWJF has a unique capacity to convene diverse and unexpected allies. Today, it's crucial to create safe spaces for exchanging ideas, grappling with challenges, finding common ground, and joining forces to work toward solutions.

That is the intent of the *Sharing Knowledge to Build a Culture of Health* conference and the book you have in hand. On these pages, you'll hear from experts across a range of sectors and political perspectives. I'm heartened that—despite their differences—these leaders share the goal of improving health for everyone in America. Amid a climate of divisiveness, this book suggests the possibility of building bridges and making a difference in people's lives.

I must recognize my predecessor, Risa Lavizzo-Mourey, for setting RWJF on this bold path of building a Culture of Health alongside new, nontraditional partners. Risa emphasized that many factors influence health—factors like education, housing, neighborhood safety, and the opportunity to earn a living wage. She pushed RWJF to convene a broad range of innovators to address such factors. During her tenure as president and chief executive officer, she did exactly that when she launched the *Sharing Knowledge* conference and this accompanying book series. I'm so pleased that Risa has contributed her expertise to Chapter 1, "Seeking Common Ground in a Time of Change."

There are many brilliant thinkers like Risa working to build a Culture of Health today and solve the puzzle of health equity. But how do we translate their knowledge into action? As an epidemiologist, I used to believe that data were enough to drive decision-making; do good research and health would improve. But here is something I learned as a former leader of the Centers for Disease Control and Prevention (CDC) and, most recently, as chief health and medical editor for ABC News: to inspire action, you have to connect first with the heart. You do that through clear, effective communication. If you can connect with the heart, the mind will usually follow.

For too long, we in public health have overly relied on the hammer of data to change behaviors, practices, and policies. One tool cannot build a house—or a Culture of Health. With that in mind, it's worth considering what "tools" we can gain from influential writers like Eugene Robinson, in order to turn research by groundbreaking scholars like Raj Chetty into better-informed policies and practices (see Chapter 2, "How Location Influences Upward Mobility and Health"). How will we harness the power of both data and narrative to inspire action?

More than ever, RWJF intends to use its voice as a tool to inform the national conversation around health and well-being. With our voice, and the voices of our grantees and partners, we will work to realize a shared vision for what a Culture of Health looks like. We will ground our communication and our action in the best research available and honestly admit what we don't know. We will connect with people where they are, and we will stand up for the fundamental principles of health and equity, even when that means risking criticism.

It's my hope that this volume will move the national conversation on health and well-being forward by sharing valuable knowledge, evidence, and real-world experiences.

—Richard E. Besser, MD
President and Chief Executive Officer,
Robert Wood Johnson Foundation

INTRODUCTION

ALONZO L. PLOUGH, PHD, MPH, MA

Chief Science Officer and Vice President, Research-Evaluation-Learning, Robert Wood Johnson Foundation

In February 2017, hundreds of researchers, policymakers, journalists, and practitioners met in Louisville, Kentucky, to explore together what it means to create an equitable society in which health and well-being characterize every aspect of life for all individuals, no matter where they live, work, go to school, or play. This lively and accessible volume from that conference is the second in the *Culture of Health* series that we hope will generate knowledge, catalyze discussion, engage new partners, and inspire action to build that equitable society.

The conference took place just three months after the conclusion of a presidential campaign that surfaced deep divisions among Americans. Declining trust in institutions long considered bedrocks of democracy also characterized the volatile political environment, with a poll by the Pew Research Center reporting public trust in the government near historic lows.[1] Only 4 percent of respondents said they trusted the federal government to do the right thing "just about always," and just 16 percent said they trusted it to do the right thing "most of the time."

Media coverage of political leaders quarreling over what constitutes a fact has added to the upheaval. These quarrels undermine meaningful discussion about important policy issues and feed a disturbing trend of questioning scientific evidence and dismissing it as a source for decision-making. Many of us wondered how we can foster health and well-being in the uncertain and contentious environment in which we find ourselves.

One way to start is by creating safe spaces for people to talk through their differences and find areas of shared interest, and that's what happened in Louisville. With a commitment to promoting honest conversation and an abiding belief that diverse populations can bridge the distances that separate them, RWJF invited people to the table from isolated rural areas as well as large urban centers, city government departments as well as federal agencies, and small community-based organizations as well as multilayered health care and insurance systems.

We had front-line practitioners, researchers, policymakers, administrators, and high-level officials there, along with people from other countries, reflecting RWJF's belief that "we are all in this together" and that the United States has much to learn from diverse experiences across this nation and around the world. Many of those we brought together work outside the health arena, including in climate change, media, start-up companies, investments, and communications.

Our approach is to embrace difference and recognize complexity, not to strive for pat answers or to expect closure. Rather than relying on rote algorithms to point us to a single solution, we are connecting multiple sources of rich data to the lived experiences of Americans, increasing our capacity to grow knowledge and improve outcomes.

While invigorating, the conversations at the conference were also tense at times. Achieving the level of health, well-being, and equity that a great nation deserves challenges all of us to step up, join forces, and take action. Many of the workshops gave us a sense of how important, and how hard, it is to move beyond words and abstract concepts to do things differently.

Equity is the power beneath and surrounding a Culture of Health, and it was a key theme throughout the meeting. Sessions about the role of race, class, place, and opportunity illustrated the effects of structural inequity on Native Americans, low-income whites living in rural areas, blacks, and other marginalized groups. While the equity goal can be a unifying force, it can also generate confusion, disagreement, and divisions that have to be confronted.

The connection between evidence and narrative was another important meeting theme. Presenters illustrated the power of tying human experience to credible research findings, reminding us that our work is about improving lives. Raj Chetty's analyses of big data told us that where we live as children affects the opportunities and choices available to us as adults, while Eugene Robinson and others offered personal stories that added immediacy and color, giving life to the data. As Richard Besser, mentions in his Foreword, data and narrative together can create a compelling story to motivate action.

Chapters in this book synthesize both the formal presentations and the vigorous discussions that followed and examine the ways in which it all connects with RWJF's Culture of Health vision. The volume proceeds as follows:

Section I, "Building a Culture of Health: The Role of Place, Race, Opportunity, and Class," draws on both data and narrative to illuminate how profoundly environment and culture can sway a life. Through provocative analyses and poignant personal stories, we gain insight into the structural disparities that are undermining the American Dream. Contributors put forward deeply contrasting philosophies about the role of government in solving problems, hinting at the struggle to reach consensus.

Section II, "Influencing Health Across Sectors," elevates the importance of involving many sectors in developing a Culture of Health. Insights from people working in fields as disparate as criminal justice, social investment, and climate change illustrate the intricate connections between health and other institutions and disciplines. Here, we demonstrate that achieving well-being is neither the sole responsibility of health professionals nor beyond the purview of any other sector.

Section III, "The Power of Collaborative Relationships," surfaces the necessity of working with people who hold very different views of the world. Value differences—called *value pluralism*—can be an essential ingredient of inclusion, but they are also a source of tension and disagreement. Stories of collaborative efforts under way in the United States and abroad ground theories of collaboration in a variety of academic and community settings.

Section IV, "On the Front Lines of Community Change," shines a light on the hard work of improving outcomes for people and communities that have long been marginalized, ignored, and treated inequitably. Even when an intervention works, further challenges arise in scaling the success for broader impact. Stories from activists on the front lines illuminate the value of admitting mistakes, learning lessons, and moving on.

Section V, "Profiles of Kentucky," portrays the conference host site in all its complexity. Remote from the "bubbles" of the coasts, Kentucky is both unique and representative. As an urban hub, Louisville has a diverse population, large employers, and a thriving tourism industry. The Appalachian region of eastern Kentucky, by contrast, sorely lacks jobs and resources and has a largely white population. Yet city and rural leaders face similar challenges in overcoming inequities, and both offer ideas that inspire.

The Epilogue offers a brief overview of the Culture of Health vision and Action Framework and RWJF's programmatic themes, as well as a look at some ways in which we, along with others, are operationalizing efforts to address health, well-being, and equity. Summary findings from a commissioned assessment of the spread and uptake of the Culture of Health vision, Action Framework, and principles of health equity provide insights around early progress and challenges.

BUILDING A CULTURE OF HEALTH

The Role of Place, Race, Opportunity, and Class

A powerful strain in American culture favors fairness. A growing share of us believes government should be responsible for ensuring health care coverage for all—60 percent said so in 2017, compared to 51 percent just a year earlier, according to the Pew Research Center.[1] Pew also found that 65 percent of Americans believe the economic system in this country "unfairly favors powerful interests."[2]

But countervailing forces are interfering with a broad commitment to equity. People who see it as a zero-sum game, with rules requiring them to give something up so others can have more, are reluctant to play. Recent polls suggest this is a prevailing attitude. One survey suggests that most white people think they get little or no advantage from their race, while only a small portion of the black population believe that to be the case.[3] Rural people generally feel that the federal government favors cities,[4] and a majority of the white working class says it does not do enough for people like them.[5]

With such schisms, is it even possible to foster a Culture of Health? Researchers, practitioners, and optimists are convinced there are opportunities for convergence, and, in this section, they point enthusiastically to bright spots where progress has been made. "Seeking Common Ground in a Time of Change" puts some of the issues in a broader context by examining the macro-level forces reshaping society, debating the proper role of government, and considering how best to build on evidence and inspire community engagement. A hunger to heal the divisions that have riven the nation almost in two is palpable in the tenor of this chapter's presentations.

"How Location Influences Upward Mobility and Health" draws on the power of both research and personal experience to describe the importance of place. By identifying the regional characteristics that make upward mobility most feasible and talking frankly about the damage done when an area lacks opportunity, the contributors make a persuasive case for building healthier communities.

"Driving Toward Racial Equity" focuses on three topics: American Indian issues, the government's power to drive change, and preterm births, mining each of them for what they can teach us about the enduring legacy of disparities. At this moment in history, we are concerned that overt racism is given voice in some quarters, and institutional racism is evident across many sectors. On the more hopeful side of the ledger is the willingness to face these challenges and confront its impact.

Throughout this section, the message comes through clearly that place, race, class, and opportunity are influential strands in the braid of challenges that lie before us. None can be addressed in isolation.

1

Seeking Common Ground in a Time of Change

MICHAEL F. CANNON, JM, MA

Director of Health Policy Studies, Cato Institute

BRUCE JAPSEN

Health Care Journalist, Forbes; Adjunct Professor, School of Journalism, University of Iowa

LEIGHTON KU, PHD, MPH

Professor and Director, Center for Health Policy Research, Milken Institute School of Public Health, George Washington University

SHIRIKI KUMANYIKA, PHD, MPH

Emeritus Professor of Epidemiology, Department of Biostatistics and Epidemiology, University of Pennsylvania

RISA LAVIZZO-MOUREY, MD, MBA

PIK Professor of Health Policy and Health Equity, University of Pennsylvania; President Emerita and Former Chief Executive Officer, Robert Wood Johnson Foundation

SARAH ROSEN WARTELL, JD

President, Urban Institute

It is hardly news that our nation is divided in many ways, and the topic of health in all its facets is as divisive as any other issue we face. Across the political spectrum, there is vigorous debate about personal responsibility, how culture influences the choices we make about health behavior, where government should (and should not) step in, and what social policies and commitments will strengthen us as a society.

This opening chapter captures some of the foundational principles of the *Sharing Knowledge to Build a Culture of Health* conference—namely, that ideological differences are welcome, that evidence is the foundation of forward movement, and that progress is not possible if we are unable even to talk to one another. Despite divergent political views and some fundamental disagreements,

> *Markets are flawed, government is flawed, our institutions are flawed. But there is ballast to be had by voice, by engagement, and dialogue with people across different parts of the system.*
> —Sara Rosen Wartell

conference speakers across the political spectrum sometimes discovered that they had arrived at similar conclusions from very different points of departure.

Among the chapter contributors are representatives of the Cato Institute and the Urban Institute, independent, not-for-profit organizations committed to shaping public policy on the basis of thoughtful, research-based analyses. They are joined by seers who look at today's uncertain and fast-changing political environment and offer educated guesses as to how the landscape for health policy might evolve in the coming years. Their shared insights and varying perspectives suggest the many points of view that will need to be considered to build an enduring Culture of Health.

Seeking Common Ground

The theme of building bridges—"deliberative processes across difference," as one speaker called it—reverberated across the conference. Too often, acknowledged Risa Lavizzo-Mourey, "we hunker down into our ideological trenches and refuse to budge" when we hear words like equity and disparities. And yet most of us share core values that transcend political lines. "I don't know anyone who doesn't want their kids to flourish, and I've never met anyone who wasn't committed to making sure that the people they love have the best chance to be healthy and get ahead and do well in all aspects of their lives," she said.

The odds are tough for some. "There are still too many places where folks find that they start behind and stay behind and too many places where people feel they've been left out or never included in the first place," said Lavizzo-Mourey. The struggles are evident in isolated rural and urban settings across the United States, places "where you see big noisy highways dividing communities, where you see toxic waste dumps next to playgrounds, and in communities where, sadly, it's easier for kids to buy drugs than to get fresh fruit."

How do we change that? True, many of us can exert some influence over our own health by choosing the salad over the brisket, the fruit over the cookies. But most of the drivers of health are far more complicated than the food that winds up on our plates. "The choices people make are so often dependent on the choices that they have, and culture is part of the way that we collectively determine the choices that people have," Lavizzo-Mourey reminded the audience.

Acknowledging that creates a framework for dialogue. "By having an honest discussion about shared values and the ways in which we collectively shape culture, we can transcend some of the political divides and get to a point where we're actually able to improve health in America," she said. Free and frank conversation, the kind that is at once essential and uncomfortable, is essential if that is to happen.

Volatility, Uncertainty, Complexity, and Ambiguity

With the *Sharing Knowledge* conference under way barely more than a month after the 2017 presidential inauguration, the unpredictable shifts that typically surround any change in leadership took on added intensity in this conference discussion. Three Washington-watchers jumped into a Town Hall–style meeting with updates, predictions, and concerns about how political appointments, budget appropriations, and the debate over the Affordable Care Act (ACA) would impact health in a world that suddenly looked very different from what most people had expected. Whatever the accuracy of their February predictions, the political ground has continued to shift.

Conference participant Lisa Simpson, MB BCh, MPH, FAAP, president and chief executive officer of Academy Health, called this a time of "VUCA"— volatility, uncertainty, complexity, and ambiguity—which is a descriptive acronym typically used by the defense sector.

Without hazarding a guess at the outcome of legislative activity, Leighton Ku noted that philosophical divisions and budget issues in Congress make it difficult to reconcile disparate health policy goals. The fate of the ACA was one of the biggest unknowns. Beyond access to health insurance, the ACA supports a broad range of research activities embedded in the Centers for Medicare and Medicaid Innovation, the Patient-Centered Outcomes Research Institute, and the Prevention Trust Fund, and their future is not clear. Ku highlighted other threatened features of the ACA, including the individual mandate, the health exchanges, and the essential benefits required of any insurance plan. Layered on top of those is a possible shift in Medicaid funding to block grants. Should the ACA be repealed or significantly overhauled, he felt it would not only push up rates of uninsurance, but also have significant consequences for health care providers, employment rates, and state and local tax revenues.

To those generally concerned about the future of important health issues, Shiriki Kumanyika cautioned against feeling powerless. "We have to keep going, no matter who is in the White House, no matter who is in the State House," she said, citing the wisdom gained through her past experiences as president of the American Public Health Association (APHA). "The closed sign is not going to be on the door. We're too important to fail."

In addition to health insurance, APHA priorities include workforce issues, health equity, and regulations designed to protect the public health, such as menu labeling and school lunch programs. With each of these under some degree of stress, strategic partnerships to carry public health messages forward become more important than ever, Kumanyika said.

Health in Context

The Urban Institute's Sarah Rosen Wartell took a step back from the postelection sense of urgency to offer a macro-level perspective. The Urban Institute houses 11 centers, focused on health, housing, communities, criminal justice, income and benefits, taxes, and other policies, giving it a unique capacity to study the origins and cross-cutting impact of a wide array of issues. Drawing on some of that work, as well as its role as a research hub for *Policies for Action,* a signature research program of RWJF, Wartell identified four contextual issues in which the Culture of Health plays out:

- **Technology and globalization are driving profound changes in the structure of the American economy.** Jobs paying mid-level wages, which once offered stability to the middle class, have been steadily eroding. This trend began before the Great Recession and has largely continued unabated. "The newer jobs that the economy is creating have on average lower pay, reduced benefits, fewer hours, and less consistent security," she said.

    This stands in marked contrast to the structural changes that have accompanied technological upheavals of the past, which generally created more employment opportunities over time. Given the body of research linking income and health outcomes, a deeper understanding of the evolving structure of the labor market is important in designing for the Culture of Health.
- **Health care costs much more in the United States than in other countries, and outcomes are much worse.** While some of this may reflect the way in which the United States delivers health care, the influence of social and economic realities is clearly a factor (see Chapter 4, "Enlisting Social Supports to Advance Health"). The resources available for the patchwork of programs that represent the U.S. safety net are low in proportion to what other wealthy countries spend, and fiscal and political realities are likely to further reduce funding.

> *Although we spend far more as a share of our economy on health than most other OECD countries, we spend less as a share of our economy on the social safety net.*
> —Sarah Rosen Wartell

That, said Wartell, creates "the imperative to figure out what brings the highest degree of return on investment for our dollar spent." As more authority devolves to the states and localities, differential models will emerge, giving social scientists opportunities to look for and test promising tools, identify what works, and figure out how they can be replicated.

- **Place matters to health.** We know instinctively that place matters to health—"where you live, the kinds of schools, whether your kids can walk to a playground, whether there's healthy food, all of those things affect your health outcome," Wartell said. Confirming instinct through research will deepen knowledge of the mechanisms by which place influences health and economic outcomes. (Raj Chetty takes a closer look at the influence of place in Chapter 2, "How Location Influences Upward Mobility and Health.")
- **As confidence in the prospects for economic mobility dims, populist pressure is building.** Wartell called these twin trends "a profound shift," noting "the idea that a rising tide is going to lift all boats has been replaced in people's minds with the idea that the tide is only rising for some people, and not for me."

   That perception largely matches reality. A Brookings Institute study showed that while most metropolitan areas had experienced net economic growth from 2009 to 2014, only 8 out of 100 regions had experienced that growth equitably.[1] Median wages fell everywhere else, and the share of workers earning extremely low wages grew in half of these areas. "We need to understand the ways that the sense of futility translates, and see if there are some shared solutions," Wartell urges.

If reason can be found for optimism, it is in the common narrative that runs through these societal trends. From rural Appalachia to the Midwestern Rust Belt to the neighborhoods of Ferguson, Missouri, growing numbers of Americans have lost faith in the nation's institutions, convinced that some people are gaming the system at the expense of others.

> *There is a rising anger, not only at wealth inequalities, but at the political system and at institutions, and a rising populism on both the left and the right.*
> —*Sarah Rosen Wartell*

While their personal experiences undermine faith in unique ways, "the fact is people believe the system doesn't work for them," said Wartell. "People are feeling a profound sense of constrained opportunity and less hope for their futures. It is a shared experience." In that common belief, she said, may lie an opportunity to pursue solutions together.

The Power of Pro-Growth Policies

Michael F. Cannon approached health and its relationship to income from a very different angle, pointing to taxation, public spending, and regulation as structural barriers to economic growth and mobility. He cited a 2009 Congressional Budget Office estimate that "tax rates would have to more than double" to keep up with current entitlement programs.[2] The "big and alarming take-away" from that finding, Cannon said, was that imposing those additional taxes would mean, decades out, that gross domestic product (GDP) would be 20 percent less than under current rates.

From his lens as a libertarian, Cannon takes a dim view of a broad range of government interventions, beginning with the transfer of resources through entitlement programs. He views that as undermining incentives for people to work or acquire new skills. Occupational licensing is another obstacle, he said, both because it makes it harder for lower skilled workers to find jobs and because medical and dental care, among other services, become costlier when they are provided by more highly trained professionals. Zoning and land-use restrictions, which can drive up housing costs, are another realm in which poor populations can be harmed by regulation.

> The high implicit marginal tax rates that result from the interaction of tax policy and welfare policy are often a barrier to upward mobility.
> —Michael F. Cannon

By contrast, Cannon noted that a large body of research demonstrates that variations in health spending don't actually affect health outcomes, and he suggested that "access to health care matters less than a lot of people think."

What does matter are institutional norms and requirements, he said. For example, state governments' unwillingness to allow dental therapists to practice at all or to allow dental hygienists an expanded scope of practice denies some patients the attention they need, Cannon believes.

Broadly speaking, Cannon views the institutional problem as one of both power and of information. "Government tends to consolidate or facilitate consolidated power," he said. "The existing payment and delivery systems in Medicare and Medicaid consolidate power in the hands of those who control the systems. They block reform, and that can have adverse effects on health."

The information problem, in turn, stems from those who are in a position to influence government decision-makers. "Most of the information the political system gets, the information it acts on, comes from the powerful, those who want to hold on to their power. When political actors use that information to make decisions and spend our money poorly, they don't get the information about how their decisions are harming people."

Across the Divide

The hope of moving forward together was clearly important to many conference speakers and participants. Land-use regulations represented one avenue of possible cooperation, given that analysts on both sides of the political divide saw their impact on housing costs as a structural barrier to mobility. As well, there seemed to be bipartisan agreement on proposals to change

> *Human beings will always make mistakes, but when they make mistakes with power, those mistakes tend to affect more people and they tend to persist longer.*
> —*Michael F. Cannon*

professional licensing requirements and scope-of-medical-practice laws to broaden access to care. More generally, consensus emerged about the value of economic growth, the importance of cost-effectiveness as criteria for promoting programs that produce greater mobility, and the imperative of creating more opportunities to realize the American Dream.

The Role of Government

None of that entirely bridges a wide philosophical and policy gap, which includes fundamental disagreements about the role of government. Long before the early-twentieth-century exposé of conditions in the meatpacking industry led to consumer protection laws and well after recent rules to further fair housing were put in place, there have been numerous efforts "to use the government as a balance to private sources of power," observed conference participant Charles Homer, former associate professor in the Department of Social and Behavioral Sciences at Harvard University's T. H. Chan School of Public Health.

Yet when David Zuckerman, manager of health care engagement for the Democracy Collaborative, asked how best to restore faith in the role of government, Cannon's reply was terse: "by having the government do less." Among other ways to shrink the public sector, he believes that repealing the ACA would help control health care costs if it were replaced with a system that allowed insurers to price coverage according to risk and made consumers more cost conscious. Wartell, however, pointed out that if risks are not pooled, many low-income people would be unable to afford their premiums and said, "You'll lower the cost of care by reducing the degree to which care and health outcomes are achieved."

Stepping back to consider Zuckerman's question more broadly, Wartell argued that as a society "we aren't comfortable with a pure market outcome" in certain arenas, such as education and health. Despite palpable skepticism about the role of government, she pointed out that "the closer government gets to them, the more people actually like it. They like their local government a lot better than they like their state government, and they like that more than the federal government. They don't like members of Congress and faceless bureaucrats . . . but they don't necessarily hate their Social Security checks."

The challenge, then, is to figure out the most efficient mechanism for engaging government, which does not tend to excel at rapid innovation and change but is often very good at implementing models once they demonstrate value. "Go local, find models of success, find disruptive innovation, and then try to leverage those with the public sector," recommended Wartell.

Sharing the Wealth

Wartell dug deeper into Cannon's argument that economic growth is generally good for health and that, as incomes rise, people make better health choices. "If there are concentrations of economic growth in a smaller number of people's hands, and the gains from the productivity of technology aren't widely shared, it's not necessarily the case that we'll get the salutary effects you ascribed to income," Wartell said. In her view, supportive policies designed to "create pathways that mitigate the effect of growing up poor," delivered with the right mix of funding flexibility and government protection, offered the best chance to make a difference in people's lives.

Cannon agreed that expanding the pie was necessary but not sufficient, and he circled back to his ideas about reducing constraints to upward mobility through various forms of deregulation. In his view, the challenge is not income inequality, per se, but whether people at the low end of the income scale are able to rise.

> The problem with only focusing on inequality is that everyone could be getting poorer and inequality could be falling.
> —Michael F. Cannon

An audience member added another element to the discussion by criticizing GDP as the primary measure of the economy because it does not differentiate among different types of spending and investment. Session moderator Bruce Japsen pointed to work on a complementary tool called the Growth Social Product, which attempts to go beyond classic economic measures to incorporate sustainability and other dimensions of well-being into the equation.

All of these issues are complicated by technological transformation and global trade and the ways in which the benefits of both are distributed across the economy. The rewards of investment currently favor capital, said Wartell. "We have to figure out ways in which labor becomes more valuable in our economy again." At the same time, trade can be something of a double-edged sword, at once generating job losses and cheaper prices for goods. Cannon quoted an official of the Obama administration as saying that if Walmart had been a government program, it would be hailed as a successful antipoverty initiative because it had done so much to stretch the consumer dollar.[3]

Evidence and Engagement

Whatever their points of intersection and divergence, the academics, policy-makers, and activists at the conference uniformly agreed that arguments need to be built on evidence. In discordant times, science matters more than ever. At a moment when "post-truth" became the Oxford English Dictionary's 2016 word of the year, Lisa Simpson called on her colleagues to "stay true to your north star of evidence." All agreed that we are in dangerous territory if opinion begins to rule over fact.

On the face of it, "post-truth"—defined as "relating to or denoting circumstances in which objective facts are less influential in shaping public opinion than appeals to emotion and personal belief"—is antithetical to science. But that does not negate the value of incorporating emotional appeal into an argument, as Richard Besser observes in his Foreword to this volume. Communications experts know that telling resonant stories—and sharing research insights to which people can relate—develops a constituency for informed policy that data alone cannot duplicate. The skill, then, is to grow stories from evidence. "There's a discipline we have to use in storytelling that isn't about picking the anecdote that says what you want," underscored Wartell. "Storytelling is about finding emblematic stories from the evidence."

Cannon, too, lamented a widespread tendency to bring bias to evidence. Worse is operating in an "evidence-free zone," as he said health policy too often tends to do. He cited the Abdul Latif Jameel Poverty Action Lab as a welcome example of an initiative designed to measure the impact of policy interventions through randomized studies.

> *I hope we can find new ways in which we can showcase our evidence and communicate about it, but hold onto those norms of rigor that we have relied upon for so long.*
> —*Sarah Rosen Wartell*

Along with evidence, engagement is essential to informed decision-making, especially when so many norms and institutions are in flux. "Stay involved, as citizens, as professionals, as scientists," urged Ku.

The oft-repeated refrain to "engage locally" reflects not only the current turmoil in Washington, but the reality that it may be easier to find common ground there. At the local level, said Wartell, "partisan divides, ideological divides are less profound and people can talk about shared experiences and converse across differences."

Attesting to a bipartisan respect for public participation, Cannon urged, "Find the policies that are holding back the people in your communities, reach out to people you wouldn't normally reach out to who might have a common interest in eliminating some of those barriers, and demand your power back."

> *Power concedes nothing*
> *without a demand.*
> *—Michael F. Cannon, quoting*
> *Frederick Douglass*

More than ever, said Kumanyika, people need to use their voices to connect and speak out, and she is encouraged to see that happening in so many venues. "People are coming out to touch each other and to experience solidarity," she said. "When you see that there are people like you, or maybe unlike you, that you're holding hands with and you're standing out in the cold with, that's really powerful."

Regardless of who joins those alliances, or what issues they are built upon, having evidence lie at their foundation is an imperative. Reasoned political debate must begin with scientific facts if we are to realize the shared hope for convergence.

How Location Influences Upward Mobility and Health

RAJ CHETTY, PHD
Professor of Economics, Stanford University; Co-Director,
Public Economics Group, National Bureau of Economic Research

JOHN FRIEDMAN, PHD
Associate Professor of Economics and International and Public Affairs, Brown University

EUGENE ROBINSON
Associate Editor and Columnist, Washington Post

Rising income inequality in the United States and its link to poor health have received significant coverage in policy circles and public conversation in recent years. Two factors in particular tug at a fundamental sense of fairness: the uneven opportunities available to children from different backgrounds and the reality that some people live longer and healthier lives than others—not because of their genetic code but because of their zip code, as the Robert Wood Johnson Foundation often says.

Place has immense power to dictate outcomes (for more insights on that topic, see Chapter 16, "A View from Appalachia"). Drawing on both big data and anecdote, the contributors to this chapter explain how environmental and cultural influences can sway a life course. Their research findings and personal experiences offer reason for concern, but also for optimism. Compelling evidence indicates that children's prospects—from earning capacity to longevity—change dramatically depending on where they live and the age at which they live there. Taking that message to heart is a powerful motivator for building the opportunity-rich environments that can transform a life's journey.

> *The American Dream is well and alive in some parts of the country, but children's chances of escaping poverty are quite poor in other parts of the country.*
> —Raj Chetty

Land of Opportunity?

The notion of the American Dream looms large in the national narrative, with its assumption that every generation will become more prosperous than the previous one. There is, granted, a certain element of myth here, and, in session discussions, one audience member sounded a note of caution. He recalled the 2016 *Sharing Knowledge* conference in Baltimore where Ta-Nehisi Coates, author of *Between the World and Me*, observed that the dream had been built in no small part on the degradation of black people.

But for all the tensions and shortcomings of American aspirations, a shared opportunity to pursue advancement remains a foundational goal. Through his Equality of Opportunity Project,[1] Raj Chetty charted the nation's progress through a data-driven research question: What is the chance that a child born to parents in the bottom fifth of the income distribution will reach the top fifth?

In the United States, there is a 7.5 percent chance of making that leap[2]; by contrast, the probability in Canada is almost double that, at 13.5 percent.[3] Comparisons with many European nations are also unfavorable: for example, in Denmark there is almost a 12 percent chance of moving from the bottom to the top quintile,[4] while in the United Kingdom that figure is 9 percent.[5]

These kinds of cross-national differences in upward mobility have generated more attention than the variation within the United States itself. Drawing on anonymous earnings records, Chetty's group measured the upward mobility of some 10 million children across 740 metropolitan and rural regions, again based on their movement from the bottom fifth to the top fifth of income.

Overlaying the findings on a U.S. map provides a strong visual portrait of opportunity or its absence. While some regions approach a 17 percent rate of upward mobility, others, such as Atlanta and Louisville, Kentucky, hover at around 5 percent (for more about the challenges in Louisville, see Chapter 15, "The Louisville Story"). In general, the Southeast and the industrial Midwest have

Often the focus of economists when thinking about inequality is labor market conditions and jobs, and that's very important. But what these data show you is that thinking about the environment in which kids are growing up is also central.
—Raj Chetty

particularly low rates of upward mobility, while parts of the East and West Coasts, as well as areas of the rural Midwest, such as Iowa and Nebraska, allow for much more movement.

Even more striking than these broad regional variations are local differentials. Zooming into a map of the Bay Area, Chetty pointed out that children growing up in San Francisco had an 18.5 percent rate of upward mobility, more than half again as high as nearby Oakland, where the figure is 11.4 percent. "Naturally, the question to us as researchers and policymakers is why upward mobility differs so much across areas, and what we might be able to do from a policy perspective or a local, social perspective to improve children's outcomes," Chetty emphasized.

The Power of the Childhood Environment

A key driver of those differences is the child-hood environment, as Chetty documented in a complex statistical study that tracked the moves of 7 million U.S. families.[6]

> *Segregation is negatively associated with children's economic opportunities.*
> —Raj Chetty

At birth, for example, a child from a low-income family in Oakland can expect to earn, on average, $30,000 per year by the age of 30. If that child had been born to a similar family in San Francisco, the expected annual income would have been $40,000. Someone from the same background who moves at age nine from Oakland to San Francisco falls about midway, earning, on average, $35,000 per year by age 30. As a child grows older, some income benefit continues to be associated with that same move, but it declines steadily, becoming essentially flat by the early 20s.

From that data, Chetty concluded that "the area in which you grow up really seems to matter for your life outcomes. . . . What these data show is that if you take a given child and move that child from Oakland to San Francisco at an earlier age, you meaningfully change that child's long-term outcome."

But the data also reveal that moving to a better environment pays off well beyond the preschool years. While scholarly work and policy prescriptions emphasize early childhood intervention, "it's not like everything is determined once you're three and then you're just off on some trajectory," confirmed Chetty. "Environment seems to matter throughout childhood."

Recipe for Success

The significant regional differences in outcome raise obvious questions: What are the defining characteristics of places that foster high mobility, and how can their attributes be replicated? Chetty described the five strongest correlations he was able

> *There's roughly a 15-year gap in life expectancy between the poorest and richest men in the United States.*
> —Raj Chetty

to identify in his research: the degree of racial segregation, the extent of income inequality, the stability of family structures, the strength of social capital, and the quality of schools.

The first four correlates can be roughly grouped as measures of connectedness, while the role of schools is a somewhat separate driver. "Places that are more connected in terms of residential structure across income groups, with higher social capital, are the kinds of places that seem to have the highest levels of upward mobility," explained Chetty.

Especially striking is the strong link to racial segregation. While segregation can be measured in many ways, "it turns out these patterns are so stark in the United States that it doesn't really matter what statistical measure you use," Chetty said. "You can just see the patterns visually."

Illustrating his point, Chetty showed neighborhood maps of Atlanta and Sacramento color-coded by race and ethnicity. Both cities have roughly the same percentage of black and Hispanic residents, but in Atlanta the populations cluster in totally different parts of the city while in Sacramento they are much more interspersed. The corresponding relationship is clear: rates of upward mobility are much higher in Sacramento.

During a later question-and-answer period, an audience member probed for the ingredients needed to "take a low-opportunity place and make it a higher-opportunity place. . . . What should we be thinking about? What is the suite of ideas that can really turn these low-opportunity places around?"

One answer is suggested in data showing significant differences in a child's chance of climbing the income ladder across neighborhoods just a few miles apart.[7] Some of these communities are "opportunity bargains," Chetty said, "in the sense that they provide really good outcomes for low-income kids but are not that much more expensive than places where Section 8 voucher holders, for example, are currently living with much lower levels of opportunity." Supporting families to use federal Section 8 vouchers to make a short-distance move could be a cost-efficient way to foster upward mobility, he suggested.

The Health Factor

Turning to health outcomes, and again demonstrating how much can be learned from big data, Chetty's research team drew on 1.4 billion records of income and mortality to measure life expectancy at age 40 for essentially everybody in the United States from 2001 to 2014.[8] The magnitude and strong upward gradient of the disparities was, he said, "quite shocking." While men in the top 1 percent of the income distribution have a life expectancy of 87.3 years, higher than any mean life expectancy in the world, those in the bottom 1 percent can expect to live only to age 72.7, roughly comparable to life expectancy in Somalia.

Local variations in broad national patterns again emerge. A chart plotting life expectancy against income in four large cities shows particularly sharp differences at the bottom of the income distribution. In New York City, for example, the poorest men are likely to live six or seven years longer than the poorest men in Detroit. (As a way of thinking about the magnitude of that difference, the Centers for Disease Control and Prevention estimates that life expectancy could be increased by somewhat more than three years if cancer were entirely eliminated as a cause of death.) Significantly, as incomes rise, life expectancy lines begin to converge, suggesting that where one lives determines the longevity of poor people more than it does those who are wealthy.

On a U.S. map, the patterns of life expectancy look similar to those of upward mobility, although they are not identical. In particular, broad swaths of the southeastern United States perform poorly on both indicators.

Informing Policy

Chetty drew out some of the public policy implications of his findings and described other work he was doing to inform action. While federal initiatives tend to dominate conversations about inequality, the heterogeneity uncovered in his data suggest the importance of local efforts, and Chetty urged the audience to think hard about how best to invest in areas of sparse opportunities.

Toward that goal, his research team is drilling further into the data, moving beyond the level of counties and metropolitan areas to analyze opportunity by Census tract and zip code. That more granular investigation, he hopes, will make it possible "to target interventions more precisely and understand exactly what works and what does not."

While again acknowledging the importance of improving childhood environments and education, Chetty warned that allocating additional resources is only a partial solution. "I'd caution that it's not just about spending more money," he said, noting that the United States already spends more on education than most other countries with better outcomes. Identifying and increasing access to high-performing schools and colleges, another avenue of research for his group, also has to be part of the equation.

Given the influence of social norms and culture on opportunity, a deeper understanding is needed about how best to foster connected communities. To inform that pathway, Chetty is looking at the relationships between local networks and poverty and well-being, drawing on Facebook data to learn how people interact and how best to leverage social capital.

Finally, he said, integrated research that examines public health and eco-nomic outcomes in tandem, rather than as distinct issues, can add to actionable knowledge. An example is a study of the Nurse-Family Partnership, an interven-tion designed to improve prenatal care through home visits (read more about this in Chapter 7, "Making the Economic Case for Population Health"). While the health benefits of the intervention have already been documented, Chetty's team is now asking whether it also has a long-term impact on a child's prospects of upward mobility.

Chetty closed his presentation with a stark chart labeled "The Fading American Dream," which showed, by the year of their birth, the percentage of children who earned more than their parents. Children born in the 1940s were virtually guaranteed to do better than their parents, but by the 1980s they had only an even chance of doing so. "This sharply declining trend has a lot to do with the issues our nation currently faces in terms of the frustration people are feeling about not being able to get ahead," he said. "One of the core challenges we all face is to figure out how we can revive the American Dream."

Americans Who Have Been Left Behind

Arguably, the 2016 presidential election was influenced by a subset of people living in regions where despair has become more prevalent than hope. But if the white working class had been largely invisible until the electoral earthquake, it represents just one of the many socioeconomic groups in urban and rural set-tings that have been bypassed by opportunity.

In recent years, a number of important works of nonfiction have put a human face on the kinds of data that Chetty and others have presented. In *Nickle and Dimed,* Barbara Ehrenreich paints a vivid picture of what it means to live as a low-wage worker in communities across America, squeezed between high rents and labor that is physically exhausting and poorly paid. *Evicted,* by Matthew Desmond, portrays families living in some of Milwaukee's poorest neighbor-hoods whose marginal economic foothold leads to repeated evictions. And in *Hillbilly Elegy,* J. D. Vance describes his journey from impoverished coal country in eastern Kentucky to Yale Law School. In the memoir, he points out that his personal story is the stunning exception in a region where loss of social capital, weakened civic institutions, and deeply depressed regional economies conspire against upward mobility.

Each of these books, and the human struggles they chronicle, "put a spot-light on a group of Americans who have been forgotten, who have been in the shadows," explained moderator Eugene Robinson. As Chetty suggested, they also undermine the core American belief that every generation will be more prosperous than the previous one.

Hillbilly Elegy, for example, offers a blunt look at the hopelessness that takes hold in a region where people's expectations are low, violence seems to the only available solution to conflict, and children have no role models pointing them toward opportunity. In large swaths of rural Appalachia, poor children are surrounded by poor adults, and neighbors are increasingly disconnected from one another. Even church attendance, which has traditionally strengthened community ties in the region, is declining.

Vance argues that understanding the outlook in some of America's most fractured communities and finding ways to reframe it requires deep insights into local culture and how it influences assumptions. While material deprivation obviously plays a significant role in the choices people make, patterns and practices that have endured for generations are also a formidable influence.

Solutions are not easy to find, but the quest can be advanced by tilting the public dialogue toward opportunity rather than dwelling on pathology. In settings like the one that nurtured J. D. Vance, changing expectations about what is possible is one of the propellants of achievement.

Rekindling the Dream

Robinson launched an audience discussion about place-based opportunity with an anecdote about his own upbringing in Orangeburg, South Carolina, where the population was roughly half black and half white. His all-black elementary school was on the campus of a historically black college, and most of his peers were the children of college professors and administrators. "I grew up thinking that black people in America were incredibly well-educated, well-traveled, urban, and sophisticated and that most white people were poor farmers who didn't go beyond a high school education," he said, laughing at a stereotype turned upside down.

Although Robinson's neighborhood was racially segregated, it was also socially and economically diverse and embraced high expectations, and the local young people generally did well. Wondering aloud whether that kind of diversity was a thing of the past, he asked, "Have we not become a more self-segregated nation by income level, by education, by political views, etc.? And does that not play a role in differentiating outcomes, perhaps a role as important as racial segregation?" Chetty agreed that mixed communities often produce better outcomes, observing that zoning and certain other urban policies, combined with the self-segregation that seems to accompany income inequality, can all contribute to greater divisions.

At the same time, encouraging people to move to communities with more opportunities carries its own complications. Many of the same settings that offer better jobs also have astronomically high housing costs that put them out of reach. And the rare people who leave their disadvantaged settings behind and manage to thrive in wealthy urban settings may deprive their communities of origins of the talent they need to build strength.

Erika Blacksher, PhD, associate professor in the Department of Bioethics and Humanities at the University of Washington School of Medicine in Seattle, pushed the discussion further into policy with her own story "of being reared in a toxic brew of domestic violence, substance abuse, legal and illegal, and chronic chaos." A first-generation high school graduate reared in a family that went from working-class poor to welfare poor, Blacksher was moved around constantly, often living with relatives. She said she had "reflected a lot about how I made my way out and how other people make their way out" and placed greater emphasis on "personal agency and personal responsibility" than many of her liberal friends tend to do.

But she was also persuaded that policy solutions are imperative, a comment that stimulated further conversation about how to broaden opportunity. While the larger forces of globalization are clearly a culprit in dragging down wages, Chetty cautioned that they do not fully explain the limits on upward mobility. If they did, he said, we would expect to see uniform consequences across the country rather than the place-based patterns he has documented. Conversely, some children growing up in low-income families in some regions do well, a finding that begs the question: What makes that possible?

The policy levers Chetty identified in his talk—reversing the disinvestment in public education, building social capital, and dismantling residential segregation—are all components of any solution. Training people for jobs that will actually exist in the near future, strengthening family networks, and confronting substance abuse and addiction also belong in the package. At a time of sea changes nationally and internationally, one audience member emphasized a framework that recognizes "there is agency at the local level."

A provocative comment about wealth and power stirred a lively discussion about the social constructs that foster their aggregation. "A lot of our culture is moving toward eroding any sort of checks and balances," he said. "And people with power keep power. How do we build a check on that?" Michael Cannon picked up on this question in his own presentation, where he called for more public participation in the policymaking process (for Cannon's perspective, see Chapter 1, "Seeking Common Ground in a Time of Change").

Robinson reminded the speaker that this is not a new problem. "I'm not sure that people with power have ever been eager to give it up. There's been a struggle to make real the promise of equality and equal opportunity that are inherent in the Declaration of Independence and the Constitution, and I think that struggle continues."

A Final Word

In drawing the discussion to a close, Robinson said that the presentations had left him with a key take-away: "local, local, local." In part, that reflects the current political moment, when it appears difficult to have a significant impact at the federal level, but it is also because many key decisions are local ones. "There is much that can be done at the state and county and municipal level," he concluded. "So let's think globally, but let's think locally as well."

Driving Toward Racial Equity

JEANNETTE R. ICKOVICS, PHD

Samuel and Liselotte Herman Professor of Social and Behavioral Sciences, Yale University School of Public Health

JULIE NELSON, MS

Director, Government Alliance on Race and Equity; Senior Vice President of Programs, Race Forward

DWAYNE PROCTOR, PHD

Senior Adviser, Robert Wood Johnson Foundation

OLIVIA ROANHORSE, MPH

Director, Native Strong, Notah Begay III Foundation

The need to confront racial injustice has been called America's "great unfinished business." Although the social and institutional milieu in which inequities are perpetuated has evolved many times over the centuries, the persistent challenge remains, as documented in both data and anecdote.

Issues of race permeated numerous sessions of the Louisville conference, and this chapter, of course, does not try to synthesize all of them. Instead, it elevates a set of presentations that call out race very specifically while positioning racial equity as part of the broader work of pursuing health for all.

Each contributor is blunt about the prevalence and impact of racism in society but optimistic about opportunities for overcoming the institutional failures that generate it. As Olivia Roanhorse describes pathways for empowering Native American communities and Julie Nelson advocates for a public sector commitment to combat institutional and structural racism, both are suggesting clear strategies for moving forward. The consequences of inaction emerge concretely in Jeannette R. Ickovics' presentation about racial disparities in preterm births, but her findings also reveal that change is possible, in this instance through the use of group prenatal care.

Dwayne Proctor introduces all of these presentations with a portrait of the "people" who represent the vast majority of this nation and whose power breathes life into the equity principles that can advance a Culture of Health.

We, the People

Hearkening back to family tradition, Proctor channeled his grandfather, a Baptist minister of the fire-and-brimstone variety, to offer a homily that touched on diversity, inclusion, and resilience:

> We, the people, who have gathered here appreciate inclusion and diversity and would like to see more of it, for we the people are not underrepresented, we are underinvited. We are undersolicited, we are underestimated, statistically speaking.
>
> We, the people, are not minorities. We are equals in all ways that matter, and when we suffer or have suffered we wish that others cared for us and treated us with the compassion and urgency that our nation directs to today's opioid epidemic.
>
> We, the people, are diverse human beings—we are women, we are men, and we like to self-identify based on our sense of self and our relationships. We the people live in hollers, cities, and suburbs, near farms, and on farms. We live in sovereign nations, and we are sovereign people.
>
> We, the people, care about our air, we care about our water, we care about our land, and we care about our nation. These are not things to us, these are our birthright.
>
> We, the people, are both young and old, and we have a variety of legal statuses. We the people are returning to our communities from prisons and wars; both are traumatic experiences and we need to be treated, clinically speaking, to help us be better people, help our families be better, and help our communities be better, because these are the things we care about. Our minds and bodies work differently, but that should not stop us from being respected or included.
>
> We, the people, understand that environments shape expectations. We the people hold a mirror up so that you can examine your own environments, your own expectations, and bring that to the table, because as much as you want to know about us, we the people want to know about you. That's authentic engagement.
>
> We, the people, understand our colleague who said that people with power keep it. We get it, because we the people believe that power belongs in

the hands of the people. We the people see ourselves as powerful, resourceful, resilient, and respectable. We do not see ourselves as vulnerable.

We, the people, want you to hear us and understand us, and we want to hear you, and we want to know about you, regardless of where we come from, or our backgrounds. We the people mean it when we say, "No change for us without us."

We, the people, know that for health equity to exist, obstacles such as poverty, social and political discrimination, and other damning systemic mechanisms that limit the potential of our people and our nation must be removed.

We, the people, are willing to fail forward with you, if we are included from the beginning to the end in your work—or, we the people will watch you fail, and you will always wonder what went wrong, if we the people aren't there with you.

We, the people, understand that charity is not equity, that equality is not equity, and that health equity requires humility on all sides. And if the eminent National Academy of Medicine can go to communities across the country, listen to them, and come up with a report that shows what systems need to change for there to be health equity in the country, we all can do that.

We all can do that, because we are the people.

A Native American Perspective

The unique history of Native Americans in the United States creates a set of challenges and opportunities that have historically distinguished indigenous communities from other communities of color. "There have been hundreds of years of systematic oppression and colonization that isn't going to come undone in one or two or three generations," said Roanhorse, who directs the Native Strong: Healthy Kids, Healthy Futures program for the Notah Begay III (NB3) Foundation.

Roanhorse is Navajo, from clans with deep connections to earth and water (she is Tó'áhání, or Near to Water Clan, born for Tódích'íi'nii or Bitter Water Clan). The NB3 Foundation, a Native-controlled nonprofit organization based on the Santa Ana Pueblo,

> *History and context are critical to understanding the current status of a people.*
> *—Olivia Roanhorse*

north of Albuquerque, New Mexico, invests in Native-led efforts to reduce childhood obesity and type 2 diabetes in Native American children. "Simply stated, incredibly difficult and complex" to execute, acknowledges Roanhorse.

Resource shortfalls are clearly part of the challenge. Despite the extreme poverty in much of Indian country, well under 1 percent of American philanthropy is focused on Native American issues (just 0.3 percent, according to one report[1]), and health is one of the lowest priorities for the available pool of funds.

Nonetheless, Native communities are working from the ground up, drawing on their rich traditions and belief systems to revitalize and build their pathways to health. An important component of NB3's mission is to showcase these approaches, connect them to other local needs, and bring Native Americans to tables where broader conversations are taking place. "That begins with communities," said Roanhorse. "An important part of our work is creating the opportunity for dialogue."

> *It's not just about inclusivity. It's also about valuing the work and seeing connections, not just within native nations but to people of color in other communities.*
>
> —Olivia Roanhorse

NB3 is sensitive both to the diversity across tribal nations and to the common threads that unite them. At a recent grantee conference, participants were asked, "What does it mean to be healthy and well in your native language?" The answers varied— *"wicozani," "wolakotu," "bimaadiziwin," "hozho"* were among them—but characteristically most tribes had just one word to express that concept, underscoring the value native communities place on a holistic (physical, mental, emotional, and spiritual) vision of health.

Unique Social Determinants

At the collaborative regional and national tables where the social determinants of health are being explored, the NB3 Foundation has identified indicators of special relevance to indigenous communities and introduced them into the larger discussion of Native American children's health. In addition to factors that are relevant to all populations, the NB3 Foundation considers the following social determinants to be core considerations[2]:

- **Access to and utilization of traditional lands.** In some cultures, the most prized assets embedded in the land are commodities like oil, timber, minerals, and real estate. But to many Native peoples, it is the priceless spiritual connection that matters much more. Rather than expressing value in terms of ownership, they view land as a "living classroom for Native nations to explain to each other what health means, what connection to food systems means," explained Roanhorse.

- **Historical trauma,** reflecting the profound emotional and psychological wounds rendered to Native peoples across generations as a result of their history of displacement and forced movement. A body of research confirms that intergenerational trauma has an impact on health outcomes over time.
- **Access to and participation in traditional cultural activities,** including the preparation and provision of food.
- **Self-determination,** built on research showing that health outcomes improve when Native nations are in control of their community and its governance. "If they take over their hospital, their education system, and they provide the culturally relevant way that they want to do the work, it has a positive association on their health," Roanhorse explained.

Indigenous Framework for Funding and Evaluation

The NB3 Foundation has made 92 grants totaling $3.2 million to 61 communities—25 to tribal nations, 36 to Native American–controlled nonprofits—since 2013. (Reflecting the depth of the need, those awards represent only 25 percent of what was requested.) These regranted funds are sourced from key funding partners, like the Robert Wood Johnson Foundation, the W. K. Kellogg Foundation, and tribal nations, including the Shakopee Mdewakanton Sioux Community in Minnesota, among other funders.

The NB3 Foundation's conviction that Native American communities are best positioned to address their own challenges alters the funding relationship. "We truly believe the solutions are in the community," explained Roanhorse. "They just need additional dollars, they need technical assistance, [and] they need professional development." But putting the grantee at the center of decision-making can admittedly be anxiety-producing to grantmakers. "If you start with that, then you have to follow them wherever they need to go. And sometimes you're not sure they are going to get there. But they will, they do, and this is the piece that I think always surprises and delights us."

The evaluation paradigm is also being changed to consider indigenous culture as a central influence on how problems are framed and tackled and how success is measured. "We clearly recognized that existing evaluation tools weren't representative of

> *It is clear to us that the role of culture is at the center of everything.*
> *—Olivia Roanhorse*

how native communities think about health," Roanhorse said. The framework for an ecosystem approach to evaluation is captured in a graphic of the traditional medicine wheel, which incorporates the mental, physical, spiritual, and emotional dimensions of health, and shows how each of those elements intersect with individual, family, community, and creation.

In consultation with Indigenous Methods Inc., and drawing on the evaluation work from the American Indian Higher Education Consortium and the Tribal Public Health Institute Feasibility Project, the NB3 Foundation developed an evaluation framework that integrates context, the gifts of Native American communities, and their view of relationships, allowing for an indigenous process to be established from the outset. "We had to change how we were talking about evaluations so that our communities felt like it was respectful and made sense from where they were coming from." This approach built on a framework developed by Marlene Brant Castellano, which describes three indigenous domains of knowledge:[3]

- **Traditional knowledge** emerges from stories and cultural engagement as passed through multiple generations of families.
- **Empirical knowledge** is learning that can be explained through observation and experimentation.
- **Revealed knowledge** is deeply intuitive.

To access these ways of learning, evaluators ask three questions at the baseline and then throughout a project's development:

- What do you see?
- What do you know?
- What do you sense or feel?

Social cohesion and connectedness is another realm in which the vantage point of Native peoples overlaps with that of other cultures while retaining unique elements. Relationships within clans, for example, are a core feature of community and extend well beyond biological ties. The indigenous model for evaluation factors in this valued asset.

Roanhorse closed her talk with brief descriptions of some of the initiatives the NB3 Foundation has supported, each built from the ground up and emphasizing Native American language, culture, and traditions. The rich and unique perspective embedded in the work is illustrated in the quote to the left of running offered by STAR School,

> *In the Navajo culture, running is about pushing yourself physically and mentally to find out more about what lives inside you. Running is prayer, a form of moving meditation and an avenue to give back to the earth that gives us so much.*
> *—STAR School Grantee*

near Flagstaff, Arizona, a public charter school based on Navajo cultural values and language.

Government as a Force for Good

While the history of Native peoples reveals that government power and authority have been applied with tragic results, they can be potent forces for positive transformation as well. With a show of hands and much laughter, virtually every audience member acknowledged, in response to questions from speaker Nelson, that they had either worked for government now or in the past or had used it. "Great," declared Nelson. "Government, in an ideal setting, should be the public sector for the public good."

Nelson worked for the city of Seattle for 23 years, including as director of its Office for Civil Rights. The length of her own tenure there surprised her because, as a young person, she thought of herself as an advocate and had assumed that change occurs when people target government, not when they work for it. Through her public service, however, she developed "a greater recognition of the leverage and power and potential" of government.

After leaving the city's employ, Nelson partnered with john a. powell to create the Government Alliance on Race & Equity (GARE), a joint project of the Center for Social Inclusion and the Haas Institute for a Fair and Inclusive Society, which powell directs. After launching in 2014 with just a handful of cities and counties, GARE now works in 150 locations in 30 states across the country to involve governments in efforts to promote increased racial equity and opportunities for all groups. Its racial equity tool supports efforts to interrupt the business-as-usual decision-making processes and self-perpetuating cycles that lead inevitably to the same outcomes.

Advancing Racial Equity: Normalize, Operationalize, Organize

As institutional and structural racism become more familiar topics of discussion in the public square, a values-driven movement has emerged to consider how those realities express themselves and what they do to us as a society. When asked what they value most, Americans inevitably call out equality and justice, however defined, and

> *There's this contradiction between what we say our values are and what we're actually achieving.*
> —*Julie Nelson*

that commitment is also deeply embedded in the nation's foundational documents. "I always like to start with the recognition that the question is less about values and more about action," commented Nelson.

Neither the legacy nor the enduring realities of racial inequity are random, emphasized Nelson. "They were intentionally created over the course of hundreds of years through laws, policies, and practices passed by government." Changing those outcomes begins with normalizing conversations about race.

That involves defining racism in its many forms, developing a shared analysis of racial equity, and being explicit about obstacles. "You have to be able to name race," insists Nelson. "We have to have the rigor and the focus to actually be able to name what it is that we are talking about so that we can develop appropriate strategies to address it. Specificity matters."

> When people say, "Let's just talk about income inequality," what is often the case is that race is an elephant in the room.
> —Julie Nelson

Once normalized, solutions need to be operationalized; that is, ideas have to get turned into action. Asking questions about who benefits and who is burdened by any given decision is a way to redirect the conversation. Collecting data is part of that process, essential to assessing needs, guiding interventions, and tracking progress. But a caveat is needed here: overreliance on data can actually stall forward motion because it does not change minds. "If people are presented with data that they disagree with, all they do is reject the data," Nelson warns.

The final step is organizing. While that term is usually thought of in the context of community, organizing can also take place within government. GARE, for example, trained 10,000 Seattle employees to integrate an explicit consideration of racial equity into policies, practices, programs, and budgets. The city now has racial equity teams and action plans in 26 departments, and GARE is promoting similar efforts in large cities like Los Angeles and New York, and in smaller places, such as Dubuque, Iowa, and Red Wing, Minnesota.

Taking on Implicit Bias

Defining and acknowledging implicit bias are essential to drive change, emphasized Nelson. Expressed indirectly and without conscious awareness, the impact of under-the-radar bias has been repeatedly documented in field after field, from public health to policing to education.

For example, despite Seattle's reputation for being progressive, research identified significant discriminatory practices in housing—almost two-thirds of landlords looking at very similar profiles of prospective renters treated whites and blacks differently.[4] Where authorities were able to establish a pattern of egregious treatment through rigorous testing, they filed charges of discrimination against the landlords. But that left a significant segment of people who did not meet legal discriminatory standards yet demonstrated a pattern of exclusionary decision-making. Often those people were sincerely upset when presented with data confirming their practice of race-based exclusions.

In response, Seattle officials worked with the Rental Housing Association of Washington to develop a set of uniform policies and practices and to conduct training for landlords. "When people know there is a potential for implicit bias and it is counter to how they define themselves, it gives us a greater ability to interrupt the response," Nelson said.

Similar training can be applied in many other fields to highlight distinctions not only between explicit and implicit bias but also between individual and institutional responses. Police officers, for example, may acknowledge that individual acts of bigotry occur on the force but might not have considered the issue from a systemwide perspective until they have an opportunity to see larger patterns in stops, arrests, and prosecutions.

Symbols are another way in which race becomes embedded in unconscious thinking. "We've got images, code words, and metaphors that are being used to trigger ideas about race, without actually naming race," explained Nelson. "Ending welfare as we know it," law-and-order rhetoric, and discussions of inner-city pathology are often ways to reference people of color without pointing directly at them.

The Art of Effective Communication

While underscoring the need for frank dialogue to root out race-based disparities, Nelson acknowledged that most people have had conversations about race that went poorly, leaving them leery of touching the topic again. After testing messages about issues such as tax policy and health care reform, the Center for Social Inclusion developed a model for more effective exchanges. Its tool kit moves people through a process of reinforcing their core values, naming the "race wedge," and identifying specific action steps to move past it.

The communication principles involved can be applied to both interpersonal conversations and policy discussions and are summarized as *affirm, counter, transform* (ACT):

- The **affirmation** is an appeal to the heart. Using health as an example, the approach would be to affirm that health depends on living in a clean environment with decent housing, good jobs, and high-quality housing. "It does not start with a mention of race. It starts with the collective value," explained Nelson.

- Next, to **counter** present-day realities, the disproportionality must be named, with an institutional explanation of the disproportionality. The statement might be "for decades, low-income communities of color have been the dumping grounds for environmental hazards. Having access to neighborhoods that support success shouldn't be determined by one's race."
- Finally, the opportunity for **transformation** is presented with specific action steps, such as supporting legislation or creating a mechanism that requires polluters to pay their fair share to create healthy communities.

> We are not going to be able to advance racial equity unless we fundamentally transform government. Those two things have to go hand in hand.
> —Julie Nelson

Nelson emphasized the tight link between advancing racial equity and an effective and inclusive democracy. The needs are urgent, she said, but the ability to change behavior lies within reach.

The Inequalities Surrounding Preterm Births

If racial injustice is a threat to democracy at a macro level, its impact is also very evident on the ground. Shifting to a specific example of how race influences health, Ickovics looked at preterm births and offered this shocking statistic: preterm births are almost 50 percent more likely to happen to black women compared to white women, across all socioeconomic backgrounds.[5]

Early delivery carries a huge price tag. There are 4 million births in the United States every year, and, at a cost of more than $111 billion, maternity care is the nation's most expensive clinical service. Despite huge medical and technical advances, 10 percent of all babies in this country are born early. That's about 1,052 infants a day, and the cost of paying for their first year of life alone exceeds $34 billion. Preterm birth is the leading cause of neonatal mortality in the United States, and virtually every organ in the body bears its lifelong scars, with enduring physical, neurological, behavioral, economic, and social consequences.[6]

Changing that demands, first, that we prioritize racial equity in women's health. Once that active choice is made, a number of proven interventions can be directed at reducing preterm birth—among them, smoking cessation, medication, family planning, optimized intervals between pregnancies, and group prenatal care. Ickovics focused on the latter strategy, which she has studied for 15 years.

The Power of Group Prenatal Care

A single twig breaks, but the bundle of twigs is strong.
                        —*Tecumseh, Shawnee leader*

Evidence-based models of group prenatal care have two components. First, they bundle social, economic, and interpersonal resources with health care to support a healthy pregnancy. Second, they bring together pregnant women of the same gestational age and their loved ones to provide mutual support. CenteringPregnancy, and a newer model that integrates a strong IT platform, Expect with Me, are the pioneers and leaders in this space.

Expect with Me's one-stop-shopping approach brings together a mix of health care services, pregnancy and birth education, and peer support in one place.[7] As the narrator on a brief video, Ickovics shared sums up, "You get more time with your provider, more knowledge, and this kind of group prenatal care lowers the risk of having a premature baby. Plus moms are healthier, especially when it comes to delivery, breastfeeding, and future pregnancies."

Two randomized controlled trials supported by the National Institutes of Health and a dissemination study funded by the United Health Foundation, have produced a compelling body of evidence about the benefits of group pre-natal care. More than 5,000 women in five cities participated in these studies. Among the findings shared at the conference:

- In a trial conducted in New Haven, Connecticut, and Atlanta, overall preterm deliveries fell by 33 percent. African-American women saw a 41 percent reduction.[8] The full study group also saw a 50 percent reduc-tion in rapid repeat pregnancies (a second pregnancy within six months after giving birth);[9] birth spacing is a known risk factor for a subsequent preterm birth.
- A study in 14 community health centers and hospitals in New York City by Ickovics and her team found that 11 percent of babies born to mothers in group care were small for their gestational age, compared to 16 percent of ba-bies born to mothers in individual care.[10]
- Women in group care had significantly less weight gain during pregnancy and lost more weight after giving birth (sustaining a 15-pound weight differ-ence after one year).[11] Excess weight during pregnancy is linked, ironically, to an increased risk of low-birthweight babies and long-term health issues, such as diabetes and hypertension, for both mother and child.
- Symptoms of depression and anxiety, which are associated with preterm birth, declined significantly among women who received group care.[12]

Results from the largest study on group prenatal care were presented for the first time at the Louisville event. A historical cohort study in Nashville, Tennessee, tracked outcomes from more than 6,400 births over 8.5 years. Women who received group prenatal care had a statistically significant—*and clinically meaningful*—reduction in risk for both preterm birth and low birth weight: 37 to 38 percent risk reduction, compared to women who received traditional individual prenatal care. These analyses also indicated that attending five or more prenatal care group sessions is optimal and feasible for improved birth outcomes.[13]

Ickovics suggested that the improved outcomes result from some combination of better knowledge and skills, changed norms about health behaviors, decreased infection, improved social support, and reduced stress and depression. The biological mechanisms at play may involve a cascade that links enhanced social support in the group setting to stress reduction and consequently a healthier endocrine milieu, cervical length, and sustained pregnancy.

Committing to Do More

Audience member Jewel Mullen, MD, MPH, MPA, former principal deputy assistant secretary for health in the U.S. Department of Health and Human Services, asked about extremely low-birthweight babies, who face the greatest lifelong developmental risks and for whom the widest racial disparities persist. Ickovics acknowledges that their mothers may be a particularly complex population to reach, but underscored the value of any extension to the length of a pregnancy. The goal, she said, is "to mobilize resources in many different ways . . . to chip away" at the problem.

A recent article in *The Nation* explicitly named racism as the answer to the title question: "What's Killing America's Black Infants?"[14] That reality, coupled with the power of the evidence, makes it urgent to "support widespread adoption, implementation, and sustainability" of the group prenatal care model, Ickovics urges. "We have evidence-based models that we need to push out, scale up, and fund in order to meet the triple aim of enhanced care, improved outcomes, and reduced costs."

Reflections on Inequity and Opportunity

An engaged audience dug further into the racial inequities that Roanhorse, Nelson, and Ickovics explored from their different vantage points. Pointing out that each presentation touched both on bringing communities together and tackling racism head on, one audience member asked how to converge those two lenses more fully.

"For me, it comes back to how we think about structural racism," answered Nelson. "There are too many examples of interventions that are done in isolation and have unintended consequences. We have to be able to break down silos and work better together."

Accentuating assets, rather than focusing on deficits, may help shift perceptions, suggested John Moon, MPP, district manager of the Community Development Department at the San Francisco Federal Reserve Bank. Moon worried that as stakeholders try to confront racial inequities, they might wind up perpetuating negative images of the communities and individuals they are trying to support. "How do you run this balance between making a case and perpetuating stereotypes?" he asked.

The strategy in the Native communities with which she works, believes Roanhorse, is to start the dialogue with the right questions, opening the door for the community to speak about its pain but also to reclaim some of its traditions. Reducing childhood obesity might be the goal, but the lead-in question might be, "What was your favorite food growing up and why?" or "What was your grandmother's favorite food and why?"

That approach can then spark a conversation about, say, the hunting and gathering practices of a grandparent. "You don't start with a negative perspective," Roanhorse explained. "You let them go where they want to go and then they will find that healing and go straight to the assets of the community."

GARE's ACT framework points in the same direction, Nelson said. "If you use a framing model that starts with the reality of what we all need, but then talks about the fact that different communities have different access to parks and healthy food, that drives an institutional response," which serves as a counterweight to a focus on individual choices as the culprit.

Picking up on this theme, another audience member suggested that one way to "switch from a negative frame to a positive frame" is to emphasize the talents being lost when populations don't have the opportunity to use their gifts fully. "We are missing the contributions that these folks can make to our society," he said.

Confronting health inequities demands both a body of evidence to inform action and a commitment to act on that evidence. Ickovics admonished the audience to act on the wisdom of Abu Bakr, a contemporary of the prophet Muhammad, who said long ago, "Without knowledge, action is useless, and knowledge without action is futile."

A Final Word

As each of the panelists documented, society's distance from true racial equity has troubling implications for population health. Bias, both explicit and

> *Let's move forward with what*
> *we know works in practice and*
> *in policy and in community*
> *engagement . . . and bring it*
> *forward to make a difference,*
> *to reduce inequities, and to*
> *promote health.*
> —*Jeannette R. Ickovics*

implicit, still thrives in America, and indeed many indicators are worsening. A rise in hate crimes and intentional acts of overt discrimination over the past few years are reminders, as Nelson observed, that "any time we make progress there is also pushback." Harder to see, but no less damaging and perhaps even more pervasive, she said, are the structures "that create and maintain racial inequities without naming race."

Outcomes in every sector—from criminal justice and education to residential segregation, the effects of climate change, and the response to natural disasters—are influenced by race. Doing what it takes to achieve greater racial equity, and in the process to advance health equity for all populations, remains the momentous task before us.

INFLUENCING HEALTH ACROSS SECTORS

The profound influence of social, economic, and environmental determinants—both on individual health and at a broader, systemic level—demands an equally broad response across many sectors. Given the disproportionate impact of health disparities on vulnerable populations, a commitment to equity reverberates throughout this section.

The chapters here draw together a diverse group of contributors—representing public health, academia, government, social service, environmental science, and criminal justice programs, as well as the insurance industry and social investing—to consider what works and how to make the necessary commitments to change. Their perspectives are those of researchers, practitioners, policymakers, and individuals who have lived experience with the issues presented.

"Enlisting Social Supports to Advance Health" reimagines how health care and social service systems can interact to improve the health of all, but especially those in greatest need. The focus is on tapping into and connecting the best parts of related systems, both locally and nationally to provide better care; improve health, social, and economic outcomes; and reduce health inequity.

"Incarceration and Health" looks at a population with the least control over their personal health and health care: adults and youths who have recently been incarcerated or remain in prison. The chapter offers sobering data and acknowledges that the connection between experiences in the health and criminal justice systems have received less attention than links between health and many other sectors. Fortunately, on-the-ground efforts to address that gap are under way.

"Resilience and Climate Change" argues that health equity, social determinants, poverty, and other key concerns cannot be addressed without attention to environmental issues. Despite a scientific consensus that climate change is real, the topic remains divisive. Contributors offer thoughtful perspectives on developing resilience, learning from past disasters, and "multisolving"—creating systemic solutions that protect the environment at the same time they build more just and healthier communities.

The section's final chapter, "Making the Economic Case for Population Health," focuses on the financial benefits of improving health across all layers of society and points out the importance of focusing cost-reduction efforts on the most expensive users of care. The contributors confront the economic effects of inequity head-on by arguing that addressing health disparities is an economically sensible approach. They also acknowledge that the long-term gains from prevention may accrue to entities other than those who make the initial investments, an outcome that can discourage financial commitments.

Integrating efforts from multiple systems, emphasizing local input and commitment, and including those whose own life experience can enrich and authenticate research and program development are all key elements of the work described in this section. The contributors build a strong case for combining the contributions of the health and nonhealth sectors to reap long-term economic benefits and improve health and well-being across American society.

4

Enlisting Social Supports to Advance Health

JO BIBBY, PHD
Director of Strategy, Health Foundation

MARIANA CHILTON, PHD, MPH
*Professor, Dornsife School of Public Health; Director, Center for
Hunger-Free Communities, Drexel University*

ANNA GOODMAN HOOVER, PHD, MA
*Assistant Professor, Department of Preventive Medicine and Environmental Health,
University of Kentucky; Co-Principal Investigator and Co-Director, National Coordinating
Center for RWJF's Systems for Action*

DAVID MELTZER, MD, PHD
*Chief, Section of Hospital Medicine; Director, Center for Health and the Social Sciences;
Chair, Committee on Clinical and Translational Science; Professor, Department of Medicine,
University of Chicago*

> *I am so poor. I am so depressed. I cannot seem to get out of it.*
> —A Philadelphia mother

Addressing the economic and social factors that influence individual and societal health and well-being requires innovative approaches that address multiple needs and systems concurrently. The work described in this chapter does just that, engaging people where they are, literally and figuratively, and then building up from there. All of it is showing early, promising results.

Two U.S.-based projects, funded by the Robert Wood Johnson Foundation's (RWJF) *Systems for Action*, take aim at components of health, economic, and social systems that can contribute to health, reduce health inequity, and foster cross-sector collaboration. *Systems for Action* is one of RWJF's signature research programs.[1] Along with *Evidence for Action, Health Data for Action,* and *Policies for Action*, it is building a broad-based body of evidence to spur, inform, and support local and national action to improve health and well-being and reduce health inequity.

An example from the United Kingdom concludes the chapter, offering a perspective on attending to economic and social determinants of health at a national level and showcasing the common threads that tie together domestic and global concerns.

Building Wealth—and Health Along With It

Through her ethnographic work with mothers of young children living in deep poverty in Philadelphia, food insecurity researcher Mariana Chilton reminds us of the health consequences of economic deprivation. Her *Building Wealth and Health Network* evaluates an endeavor to integrate the delivery of medical care, mental health services, cash assistance, and employment support for caregivers of young children by aligning Temporary Assistance for Needy Families (TANF) and Medicaid behavioral health services. Many of these caregivers were exposed to trauma, abuse, and neglect during their own childhoods.

TANF is a federal program that provides block grants to states to design and operate programs that help needy families achieve self-sufficiency. While TANF has other purposes, "the ultimate goal for TANF is to get people into the labor force, and that is the only goal by which states are actually measured," said Chilton.

Chilton's team seeks to understand how Medicaid and TANF can be merged to help build a Culture of Health within the program and promote self-sufficiency. The overarching research question is, "How do we reduce health disparities through merging or aligning systems?"

Witnesses to Hunger

The *Building Wealth and Health Network* emerged from Chilton's work in food insecurity and her understanding of the role of toxic stress in cognitive, social, and emotional development. One of her food insecurity projects is *Witnesses to Hunger*, which originated in Philadelphia in 2008. It currently includes more than 100 participants in Baltimore; Boston; Camden, New Jersey; New Haven, Connecticut; Philadelphia; and Washington.

"The idea behind *Witnesses to Hunger* is that the people who are experiencing hunger and poverty are the ones who should be framing the conversation," Chilton explained. The women are given direct access to legislators so that they can be their own advocates. Working together has fostered an experience of connectedness and a sense of power among the women.

Participants photograph elements of their lives to illustrate the experience of hunger and trying to feed a family. Chilton described her charge to participants in the program like this: "I'm interested in food, grocery stores, and food stamps, but tell me what's important to you." What came back were "profound" photos related to violence, housing, and isolation, with depression a particular theme. Many illustrated stark systemic failings, with captions like:

- "The help is out there but I can't get to it" (no phone and no way to connect with a case worker).
- "I call this graduation to the same poor wages" (TANF training programs that don't lead to better jobs).

TANF, Supplemental Nutrition Assistance Program (SNAP), and meager wages from TANF-approved jobs are not enough to support a family, so the women have "side hustles," small businesses such as doing hair or nails or housecleaning. They don't tell their caseworkers because it would be reportable income and their TANF benefits would decrease; but if the caseworker learned about it, they would be cut off immediately for fraud. In Chilton's view, the women are entrepreneurs. "Entrepreneurship in any other setting would be celebrated. Yet within the frame of TANF, entrepreneur caregivers are considered criminals."

> *Welfare is like a chain.*
> —*A Philadelphia mother*

Chilton came to realize that income alone is not enough to provide financial security. People also need to build their asset base so that they have resources to cover emergencies and outlays such as security deposits and savings. But TANF's asset limits "keep people unbanked" and "out of the financial mainstream" because a bank account would make their small and inconsistent income visible.

Research has shown that people receiving TANF have major barriers to work, including very high rates of depression, significant exposure to violence, and frequently sick children as a result of food insecurity and poor housing.[2] The opportunity to promote physical and mental health by increasing a family's financial security became clear to Chilton. "All these things can keep kids healthy, keep them out of the emergency room."

Toxic Stress

The experience of abuse, homelessness, hunger, and other adversity creates a level of "toxic stress" for young children that has major impacts on cognitive, social, and

> *There is really no Culture of Health in TANF.*
> —*Mariana Chilton*

emotional development; school performance; and workforce success, with life-long consequences. Toxic stress "can actually alter the structure of the brain," noted Chilton.

Adverse childhood experiences (ACEs; a term that originated in research pi-oneered by Vincent J. Felitti and Robert Anda in 1998[3]) have been linked to chronic diseases such as cardiovascular disease and diabetes and to premature mortality. ACEs include physical or emotional abuse or neglect, sexual abuse, parental separation or divorce, exposure to domestic violence or substance abuse, household mental illness, and incarceration of a household member.

Chilton was particularly interested in depression and the limited educational and economic achievements of low-income women. Her work takes a "two-generation approach"—"if you want to help a child avoid toxic stress, you have to work with the parents, who may have experienced a lot of toxic stress when they were children."

Trauma-informed practice is a core component of the programs to assist low-income mothers and their children that she believes has value. In this model, recognizing and responding to the signs of trauma-related behavior are central to the way programs, practices, and policies are created, as is ensuring that they do not "retraumatize the people you're working with."

Psychiatrist Sandra L. Bloom, MD, developed, at Drexel University, the Sanctuary Model for the treatment of trauma-related emotional disorders. Bloom has found that people who have experienced severe trauma have a very difficult time managing their emotions, including addressing grief and loss, thinking about the future, and setting goals.

Chilton's work with *Witnesses to Hunger*, coupled with Bloom's experience with traumatized women and the recognition that trauma-informed practice is critical, led to thinking about systems change and the development of the *Building Wealth and Health Network*.

The Building Wealth and Health Network

The *Building Wealth and Health Network*[4] is a multipart, peer-learning program for individuals with little or no income. A 16-week curriculum combines finan-cial education with the trauma-informed Sanctuary Model. Topics cover basic fundamentals about managing finances, such as reasons for having a savings ac-count, "paying yourself first," credit scores and how to improve them, and saving part of the earned income tax credit.

The program includes a savings account for each participant at a federal credit union and matches participant savings up to $5 per week in the hope that they might be able to save about $500 per year, an amount well under the TANF asset limit. Participants are considered members, and both group and individual savings goals are established.

"There is a sense of connectedness," Chilton stressed. "With standard TANF, it's all business, serious, and according to participants, no fun. Whenever you come to the Network, there is a lot of fun to be had, a lot of love and joy to help counteract the depression and stress of poverty."

A Network Advisory Council, whose members have completed the program and receive an honorarium to serve a one-year term, provides feedback and guidance on programming, evaluation, and dissemination.

Evaluating the Network

Chilton and colleagues conducted a randomized controlled trial of the *Building Wealth and Health Network* with 103 TANF recipients who were mandated to work. Participants were organized into a control group, a partial intervention group that received financial education and the matched savings account, and a full intervention group that received trauma-informed peer support services in addition to the education and savings account.

The researchers collected data on a series of measures at baseline and every three months afterward for 15 months. Measures included income, education, "under the table" work, financial well-being, asset savings, economic insecurity (a bundle of hardships that include food, housing, and energy insecurity), and maternal and child development. They also assessed depression in the mothers and cognitive, social, and emotional development, hospitalizations, and other factors in the children.

Baseline data revealed the severe hardships the women face: very high rates of housing insecurity (67 percent), food insecurity (59 percent), and depression (55 percent). Thirty-nine percent reported four or more ACEs, making them an especially vulnerable group.

Unlike other TANF-related programs, *Building Wealth and Health Network* members do not receive employment coaching, which concerned state officials who approved the experiment. Despite their worry, many of the program's findings were positive. Over the course of 15 months,

- Depression decreased for the full intervention group. By contrast, depression increased after 9–15 months in both the control and partial intervention groups.
- Based on measures of economic insecurity, hardship decreased for the partial and full intervention groups by 12 months, but increased by 15 months. Chilton speculated that more intensive services might be needed.

- Employment increased substantially by 12 months for all groups, then began to decrease in the control and partial groups while continuing to increase for the full intervention group. Income for the full intervention group also increased to the end of the intervention.

Network Redesign

Under the *Systems for Action* grant, Chilton and colleagues redesigned the *Building Wealth and Health Network*, shortening the timeframe and strengthening the curriculum, in order to look at

- Effects of trauma-informed peer support built into education and training on health and economic security.
- Cost savings to Medicaid and TANF. Since the full intervention appeared to reduce depression and increase income and employment (even without the employment coaching that other TANF programs include), researchers sought to make a case for linking these systems.
- Engagement of multiple stakeholders to promote a Culture of Health in anti-poverty programming through strategic public dissemination.

Two cohorts (94 caregivers of children under age six) have completed 12 months under the redesign. A control group will be created from an administrative dataset.

Preliminary results at 12 months were encouraging:

- Food security, about 50 percent at baseline overall, increased to 68 percent, despite a dip at nine months. Members with four or more ACEs increased their food security from 38 percent to 62 percent. "We were able to help the most severely traumatized individuals, which was our goal," said Chilton.
- Caregiver health improved significantly by 12 months for the cohorts overall and for those with four or more ACEs (after declining through nine months).
- Depression declined overall. In particular, the group with four or more ACEs showed a significant decrease by 12 months (from 79 percent at baseline to 46 percent) after some interim volatility.
- Employment increased significantly from baseline (18 percent overall and 21 percent for those with four or more ACEs) to 12 months (55 percent and 54 percent, respectively).
- Program members were much more likely to have checking and savings accounts by 12 months than at baseline. For example, only 28 percent of those

with four or more ACEs had savings accounts at baseline while 92 percent had such accounts at 12 months. Checking accounts for that group increased from 50 to 77 percent.

Next Steps in Integrating Medicaid Into the Building
Wealth and Health Network

Current work with the Network is grant-funded, and Chilton acknowledged that TANF officials "are not yet open to focusing primarily on behavioral health issues or loosening work requirements." She hopes that demonstrating how trauma is fundamental to the lives of the people involved and that a trauma-informed approach can reduce depression will earn support for pulling in Medicaid behavioral health.

"The idea is to help TANF become a trauma-informed system. Right now it's a traumatizing system with lots of hypervigilance by the state on all participating families," said Chilton. Doing trauma-informed work within TANF has been "a big leap outside health care," she acknowledged.

Fostering Comprehensive Care, Community, and Culture

In other work designed to improve health outcomes and overall well-being in the most vulnerable populations and to control health care costs, David Meltzer and colleagues at the University of Chicago focused on patients at increased risk of hospitalization.

The national need to control health care costs frames Meltzer's work. While 25 percent of Medicare beneficiaries account for 85 percent of costs, he noted, "the converse is critical: the bottom 75 percent is not driving health care expenditures. Efforts that target those people are going to have an extremely hard time recouping their costs, much less reducing health care costs." In his view, the focus must be on the high utilizers of care.

Meltzer referenced a number of ideas that have health-related merit but may not substantially shrink costs: prevention, comparative effectiveness research, care integration, and bundling capitation and accountable care organizations ("particularly challenging for the most vulnerable patients where most of the savings are").

So, he wondered, "What do you actually do on the ground to make these things work and improve patient outcomes?"

Hospitalists and High Utilizers

Concentrating on patients with high rates of health care utilization, especially hospitalization, Meltzer investigated the role and impact of hospitalists—physicians who take over care for patients after they are admitted to the hospital. The specialty developed in the mid-1990s, and there are 30,000 hospitalists in the United States today.

This specialization allows for increased expertise, inpatient focus, and clearer physician hospital presence. But it also contributes to the loss of the doctor–patient relationship, requires coordination among physicians, and can lead to communication errors.

Meltzer came to believe the hospitalist model actually grew to meet the needs of ambulatory care, not those of hospitals. As medical practice changed and physicians were seeing fewer hospitalized patients, they felt their time could be better spent seeing multiple patients in the clinic rather than following them in the hospital.

"There are a lot of reasons to worry that that is a big loss," he said. "There is a rich literature on the value of the doctor–patient relationship" that emphasizes trust, communication between doctor and patient, and patient knowledge. Studies also show reduced costs and fewer emergency hospitalizations, shorter hospital stays, and lower intensive care unit visits among patients who have a long-term relationship with their primary care provider.

His conclusion: "Discontinuity is harmful and costly, especially for complex patients, and it raises the question of whether better care coordination of inpatient and outpatient care could improve outcomes." Meltzer and his colleagues developed a strategy "to improve care by making it possible for high utilizers to be a part of a meaningful, durable relationship."

This new practice model focuses on patients at the highest risk of hospitalization. Because their practice is devoted entirely to that population, hospitalists can see multiple patients during hospital rounds while also serving in a clinic that is small enough to allow adequate time with these patients.

The advantages are many, Meltzer said. Frequently hospitalized patients can choose their own doctor who treats them in both settings, a valuable continuity that reduces testing and treatment. For physicians, it is a practical approach that affords them significant hospital experience and presence.

The Center for Medicare and Medicaid Innovation (CMMI) funded Meltzer and his team to study whether this model would work. They focused on high-cost patients who are hospitalized at least 10 days a year, at a cost of about $100,000. With a small practice size of about 200 patients, a tight, interdisciplinary team (five physicians, an advanced practice nurse, an RN, an LPN, a social worker, and a clinic coordinator) can organize care around patient needs. The key element of the model is improving the doctor–patient relationship.

The team conducted a 2,000-person randomized controlled trial with the triple aims of better care, better health, and lower costs. They have found "very promising evidence" of improved patient satisfaction and some measures of health, as well as evidence of lower costs that should make the model sustainable and attractive to payers.

Longer term funding from CMMI allows the team to continue studying this model and to address financial sustainability by developing both fee-for-service and risk-based contracts. The team is also developing partnerships with other interested institutions, including five in the United States and one overseas.

Expanding Approaches to Comprehensive Care

Despite the promise of the model, about 30 percent of participating patients do not fully engage (e.g., by not making appointments, taking medications properly, or seeking appropriate treatment), thus reducing the opportunity to provide efficient care, generate better health, and lower costs. Age and health status are not the defining characteristics of this subgroup, but they do tend to have lower incomes and less social support.

When asked why they do not engage, patients mention barriers such as transportation or mood. Deeper emotional and psychological components—such as depression, not wanting to be bothered, or preferring to do something else—often emerge on closer look. While these patients have access to resources, they are not using them.

In response, Meltzer and colleagues built the *Comprehensive Care, Community, and Culture Program* to include three elements.

- **Assessment of unmet social needs.** Using a Health Leads questionnaire, patient needs are assessed in 17 domains, such as food, housing, employment, and engaging in activities. About half have few or no unmet needs, while the other half have multiple and often interrelated unmet needs. Thirty percent of the total group have more than five unmet needs.

> *You can't just pick one of these things, you've got to pick all of them if you really want this to work.*
> —David Meltzer

- **Community Health Worker Program.** Community health workers are used to engage patients, understand and address their unmet social needs, help them navigate the system, and connect them to economic and other resources—"pull them out of their homes, connect them with the teams."

These workers do not focus on illness but are instead tightly linked to the care team and participate in daily rounds.

- **Artful Living Program.** A wide variety of resources are built into the clinic day to connect patients with the team: music, art, theater, movies, books, speakers, exercise, cooking, even revenue-generating crafts. A goal is "to promote self-efficacy and to explore and share values that enhance life and health."

The Pilot

With *Systems for Action* funding, 100 people are enrolled in a randomized controlled trial of the program, again with the triple aim of better care, better health, and lower costs, as well as what Meltzer calls "goal attainment—asking patients what's important to them and seeing whether we can help them achieve that."

By talking with patient and faculty advisory groups and asking patients directly about what they want, researchers have found "the key thing is the emotional overtone and the need for relationships." While specific interests have surfaced, with cooking taking first place, the greatest obstacle to engagement is psychological. One patient explicitly acknowledged this by asking and answering a question: "What's the biggest barrier? Me."

The pilot study seeks to show savings and efficiencies, such as reducing no-shows. To build the business case for payers and health systems and to keep costs low, the team also optimizes the use of existing community resources and mines various philanthropic sources, such as small donors and arts foundations.

"It's a fun program to work on, and we're very much in the early stages," said Meltzer. "But I'm hopeful that we can now transit this relationship we've built with patients around medical care into meeting some of their other needs."

Changing the Global Conversation: Good Health as an Asset

Imagine if global conversations about health could pivot from "ill health as a burden" to "good health as an asset." Imagine if governments were to create national policies that supported everyone's opportunities for a healthy life. And imagine if local actions could address glaring discrepancies in individual opportunities for a healthy life—not only access to health care, but equity in education, employment, housing, healthy food, and social connections.

These are long-term strategic goals of the Health Foundation, an independent charity committed to bringing about better health and health care for people in the United Kingdom. First introduced in 2017, these goals recognize that "the greatest influences on our well-being and health are factors such as education, employment, housing, and the extent to which community facilitates health habits and social connection," said the foundation's Jo Bibby.

"While equipping health care systems to provide safe, timely, and effective care is as important as ever," Bibby added, "this is far from sufficient to improve people's health. Good health is an asset. It is necessary for a prosperous and flourishing society."

Asking Questions, Listening Carefully

For 18 months beginning in 2015, Bibby researched and developed the Health Foundation's strategy to improve health through the framework of social and economic determinants. She talked to experts about how to bring about the necessary changes, debated with colleagues about how best to adopt a systems approach that worked across sectors, and listened intently to ordinary people as they discussed the factors and outcomes that impacted their health.

The goal was to distill these conversations into guiding principles. While the role of social and economic determinants is "obvious to those in the public health community," she said, "others aren't necessarily aware that health care only contributes 10 to 20 percent of your health. We think reinforcing this is important."

One question was harder to answer than Bibby expected: In whose interest is good health? While every sector has the potential to contribute to improving health, few see it as their role or in their interests. Beyond the individual, said Bibby, "It is clear that it's in *all* our interests to have good health if we want a flourishing society."

Difficult, too, was how to grapple with the United Kingdom's National Health Service (NHS), one of the world's largest publicly funded health services. According to Bibby, "We have this wonderful heath care system but it doesn't necessarily have creating good health as its core driver. In a finite resource envelope, there is a risk that the NHS's emphasis on treating sickness and disease is at the expense of the services and systems that probably would be more effective in creating long-term health."

The question is: How do we make the case for the wider economic and social value of health and help people think about health as part of core infrastructure, like transportation, housing, or energy? "If we started to think of health in those terms, it would create some different financial incentives and possibilities," Bibby suggested, wondering how to encourage people to think that any money spent—whether by charity, business, or government—has an impact on long-term health outcomes.

Healthy Lives in the United Kingdom

To help answer these questions, the Health Foundation released its healthy lives strategy in January 2017.[5] Its intent is to change the conversation to focus on health as an asset, to promote national policies that support everyone's potential for a healthy life, and to encourage local actions to address differences in opportunities.

The report notes, "Although the health of the U.K. population has seen improvements in the last 50 years, we nevertheless face a formidable burden of preventable disease. The shortcomings of a system that has focused disproportionately on treating disease when it arises, rather than investing in actions that maintain health over the life course, is becoming more visible."

The strategic plan includes key action steps:

- **Adopting a social determinants approach to improving health,** a model that seeks to identify the "causes of the causes." For example, a child who develops asthma due to poor housing and lack of access to green space and the increased risk of chronic stress and cardiovascular disease on a low-paid, temporary worker point to unequal social and economic conditions.
- **Seeing health as an asset.** This view defines a "healthy person" not as someone free from disease but as someone with the opportunity for meaningful work, secure housing, stable relationships, high self-esteem, and healthy habits. Understanding health in these terms helps to define the lack of employment opportunity and limited access to affordable housing as health problems and points to the need for actions that promote the conditions for good health.
- **Taking a systems approach** that looks to wider economic and social conditions that impact individual health.
- **Working across sectors** in health care, government, education, and business to maintain and improve health at national and local levels.

Moving Forward, Taking Action

Understanding the complex relationships between an individual's health and the landscape of economic and social determinants of health is at the forefront of RWJF's relationship with the Health Foundation. Through RWJF's global health program, the two foundations are working together to change the international conversation about health.

It's hard to find a sector that doesn't have a bearing on our health.
—Healthy Lives for People in the UK, 2017

RWJF's Alonzo Plough observed that international and local perspectives are often quite similar. Plough said that the challenges facing rural communities in Kentucky (see Chapter 16, "A View from Appalachia") are "not dissimilar to dynamics in the United Kingdom. This worsening of economic and health status of marginalized, working-class white populations in the United Kingdom is just as evident."

Inspired by the work of RWJF to reframe its approaches through the Culture of Health lens, the Health Foundation has taken steps to put its strategic plan into action.

First on the agenda has been to change the conversation from "ill health as a burden" to "good health as an asset." "Fundamentally, this is not an evidence problem; it's a communications problem," said Bibby. "We want to follow RWJF's lead in the way they've invested in communications around getting these messages out beyond the public health community and, hopefully, getting that message to stick."

The Health Foundation is also promoting national policies that support everyone's opportunities for a healthy life and research to support the value of health to economic and social development, rather than just emphasizing the cost of ill health. And, motivated by RWJF's *County Health Rankings & Roadmaps*, an initiative that measures the health of nearly all U.S. counties and ranks them within states, the Health Foundation has explored ways to support local action and evidence while becoming what Bibby calls a "main integrator of information."

Spreading Innovation

The promising results of the initiatives described here raise an obvious question: How can such innovations be spread more broadly for wider impact?

One strategy is to foster their appeal across the ideological spectrum. In Pennsylvania, the goal of giving power back to the individual and the group resonated with a very conservative Republican governor who authorized the *Building Wealth and Health Network* as an official demonstration project in the state's Department of Human Services.

Chilton noted that congressional interest in blending funding streams and letting states decide how to invest the resources created an opportunity for integrating funding systems. Private investment, perhaps through social impact bonds, may also help programs expand and scale. "In the end it will save the government a lot of money, and it reduces the need for more government intervention," she said.

Key elements in spreading a social program, Meltzer added, include understanding how it works in different settings, compelling data, adaptability in different payment environments ("critical to appealing across the political spectrum"), and finding new and easier ways to implement the model.

Compelling evidence for the value of integrated budgeting across health care and social services is also key, sending a message that "we can't afford not to do this." But Meltzer cautioned that great ideas don't always work so smoothly in practice, so care must be taken in making policy changes that affect people's lives.

"There are so many people in the system talking about the same thing, but they come at it from a poverty lens or from a public health lens," said Jo Bibby. "We're starting to explore having some sort of integrator function that curates and translates all of the evidence and data that's out there to amplify it for a wider audience to support action."

As Anna Goodman Hoover noted, "Findings from these and other studies better position us to address systemically the economic and social determinants that help drive health status. Together, we're developing a research portfolio that tells a compelling story and can help drive larger scale experimentation and innovation to improve health and well-being, particularly among our most vulnerable populations."

Incarceration and Health

GEORGE GALVIS, MCP

Cofounder and Executive Director, Communities United for Restorative Youth Justice

KAREN LASH, JD

Practitioner in Residence, Department of Justice, Law and Criminology, American University

ANNA STEINER, MPH, MSW

Program Manager, Transitions Clinic Network

Compared with the health benefits of having a job, a safe place to sleep, and clean air to breathe, the connections between prisons and health equity are not always readily apparent. Who understands, for instance, how health care inequalities and incarceration intersect, both within and beyond prison walls? That charging youths as adults leads to negative health impacts? Or that connecting criminal justice with health system reforms benefits a broad population?

The contributors to this chapter address all of these issues as they explore the links between criminal justice and health and personalize the incarceration experience. With stark data that show individuals facing an increased risk of death in the first two weeks after their release, the authors underscore the importance of programs designed to help newly released individuals navigate the health care system outside prison. And by identifying critical intersections between incarceration and health, they underscore existing inequities in both systems and highlight the imperative for reform.

Inside Adult Prisons: Portraits of Disparities and Despair

Individuals imprisoned in the United States are marginalized and often unknown to the world outside, yet their numbers are large, according to Anna Steiner, program manager at Transitions Clinic Network, a national system of clinics that provide health care and reintegration services to individuals re-turning to the community following incarceration. Much of Steiner's career has involved efforts to remove systemic and institutional barriers to people with criminal records, with an emphasis on addressing the deep disparities and health inequalities among formerly incarcerated individuals.

More than 2.2 million individuals are in U.S. prisons—the highest per capita incarceration rate in the world and a 500 percent increase in the past 40 years.[1] This means that 620 per 100,000 adults are imprisoned here, compared to 114 per 100,000 in Canada, and 101 per 100,000 in France.[2] And there are stark disparities in who gets incarcerated in the United States. The likelihood of life-time imprisonment is 1 in 17 for white men, 1 in 6 for Latinos, and 1 in 3 for black men.

Though movies and television often give the impression that those in prison are young and healthy, they actually tend to be older and sicker than the general population:

- Nearly 85 percent of incarcerated individuals have a chronic medical con-dition, including diabetes, hypertension, asthma, hepatitis C, substance use disorders, and mental health disorders. One recent report noted that incar-cerated people experience disproportionate rates of communicable disease, chronic health conditions, and mortality compared to the general U.S. popu-lation.[3] Some of these health problems are generated by prison conditions—overcrowding, loss of privacy, violence, isolation, imposed rigid routines, stress of navigating social hierarchies, and lack of social support.
- The prison population is aging. "Due to mass incarceration, harsher prison terms, and the war on drugs we're seeing people growing old in prison," said Steiner.
- Rates of substance use disorders and mental illness are significantly higher in prison than in the general population. An estimated 50 percent of state prison populations[4] and 68 percent of those in county jails[5] have a diagnosable sub-stance use disorder, compared to 9 percent of the general population. This leads some to call prisons and jails the "new mental institutions," Steiner said.

  To help the audience visualize the limits of mental health care in prisons, she showed a photograph of a group therapy session—with men sitting alone inside individual, heavily barricaded and locked cages, lined up side by side in a semicircle. Asked Steiner, incredulously, "How therapeutic do you think this is?"

Steiner noted that while health care in prison is a constitutional right guar-anteed by the Eighth Amendment, "that does not mean it is adequate. The prison environment can exacerbate poor health. Things like confidentiality, autonomy, and privacy are compromised. The system breeds passivity, and individuals may be penalized if they try to actively participate in their own care."

Distinct barriers exist when incarcerated individuals do try to access health care in prison. Some states require imprisoned individuals to write a grievance to see a doctor, a request that is then evaluated first by a correctional officer and then by a nurse. Prisoners often must pay a $5 copay for a visit, which can be the equivalent of four days' worth of prison work.

If they do receive health care, it is often inadequate. In one chilling story, a man experiencing chest pain submitted his request to see a doctor, who gave him an antacid before sending him back to his cell. Later that night, the man was found dead of a heart attack. He had written his wife a note that said, "I think I'm having a heart attack and I tried to get care. If I don't see you again, I love you."

Outside Prison: Disparities Continue, Recidivism Is High

These people really exit one broken system and enter another one.
—Anna Steiner

Almost everyone in prison ultimately goes home—and most of those released are incarcerated again. According to Steiner, 95 percent of those incarcerated will eventually be released into the community,[6] and 67 percent of them go back to prison within three years.[7] This means that a staggering 11 million individuals cycle in and out of the prison system annually.[8]

The health-related challenges for incarcerated individuals upon release are significant. As Steiner explained,

- Prisoners receive no discharge planning when they leave and no information about how to obtain medications or health care.
- There are no instructions for coping with the lack of medical insurance on the outside or with lapses in Medicaid or Medicare coverage.
- Prior to release, there is no review of the barriers they will face gaining access to basic needs like food, housing, and employment. When people are released, "they face what is called the 'collateral consequences' of incarceration: policies or laws that are used to punish people even after they've completed their time in prison." Prime examples are restrictions on Section 8 housing and benefits from the Supplemental Nutrition Assistance Program (SNAP) for drug felons.

Karen Lash offered what she called a "classic example" of trying to cope after release from prison: "You have a criminal record, and that means you're having a hard time getting a job so you don't have income. How can you possibly improve your health? In this scenario, perhaps a legal aid attorney can step in, have a criminal record expunged or sealed, and possibly reinstate a driver's license that was revoked as a condition of parole. Only then can you get a job, make money, take care of yourself, and have a much better chance of getting healthy."

The nonexistent preparation for life after prison has dire and immediate consequences for many. "It's probably no surprise that people get sicker when they come out and in fact are more likely to die," Lash said. A 2007 study published by the *New England Journal of Medicine* reported that previously incarcerated individuals have 12 times the risk of death in the first two weeks after their release from prison compared to the general population.[9] The leading causes of death include drug overdoses, cardiovascular disease, homicide, suicide, and cancer.

> *This is a public health crisis. There are things that we could be preventing and managing.*
> —Anna Steiner

Transitions Clinic Network: Fighting for Change

When people are released from prison, they face what Steiner described as "barriers to care engagement" that are not unlike the health care barriers they experienced while incarcerated.

Simply stated, the health system as a whole is not equipped to help these high-need individuals deal with mental health and substance use disorders or the complex traumas they experienced before and during incarceration.

Even if such health systems existed, Steiner noted that individuals post-incarceration have little experience trying to navigate complex systems, which can be difficult for anyone to access. "The major systematic issue is that we have siloed systems," she said, "correctional, community-based services, health care. They don't communicate and collaborate, which results in even more barriers to individuals receiving the care and help they need."

For the post-incarcerated community, Steiner emphasized the need to shift the paradigm from a traditional, primary care model to a comprehensive model of care that is supportive, addresses social determinants of health, and works across sectors within communities.

Transitions Clinic Network does exactly that. Founded in 2006 by Emily Wang, MD, and Clemens Hong, MD, this national network of 17 clinics in eight states and Puerto Rico serves more than 3,000 patients recently released from prison. Based on the premise that the people closest to the problem are also closest to the solution, each clinic employs a community health worker with a history of incarceration as part of its clinical team.

Transitions Clinics are located in communities most impacted by incarceration and are part of existing health care clinics. This concept was extremely important to community advisory board members because it allows patients to be integrated into community care and not treated punitively. (Shira Shavit, MD, executive director of Transitions Clinic Network, was a Robert Wood Johnson Foundation [RWJF] *Community Health Leader* recipient in 2010.)

The Community Health Worker

The linchpin in the whole concept, said Steiner, is the community health worker who supports individuals as they navigate the world beyond incarceration. Community health workers help make and sustain key collaborations between primary care and individuals within two weeks of their release and help them manage chronic health issues. They promote behavioral health services integration, help ensure parole and probation contacts, and foster reentry support with existing community organizations that deal with everything from housing and employment to social challenges.

As she shared pictures of two community health workers, Steiner illustrated just how broad their role can be. There's Ron, serving as an interpreter between a physician and a patient in a clinic examination room before moving on to greet patients in the larger waiting room to ensure that they feel comfortable. And there's Juanita, bringing food to a Transitions Clinic participant who couldn't make it to a food bank.

> *One of the great things about the community health workers is they are really able to transcend the static walls of the clinic. They open up the walls of the clinic to bring in some nontraditional, reentry service providers.*
> —Anna Steiner

Improved Reentry and Health Outcomes

But does the model work? A 2010 randomized controlled trial of the Transitions Clinic model, using electronic health records and county jail data, showed that it improved reentry and health outcomes.[10] Consider:

- Individuals who received care at Transitions Clinic Network were less likely to use an emergency room in a 12-month period, resulting in an average cost savings of $912 per year, per person, compared to a traditional clinic.

- Recently released patients who attend two or more visits to their assigned clinics are less likely to go back to prison than those in the community.
- Community health workers are successful in engaging the post-incarcerated community in care.

"Success to us means that people want to engage and use our services, that they come back, that they reintegrate successfully into the community and continue to be engaged with us," Steiner said. Based on the study results, the Transitions Clinic Network received a three-year Health Care Innovation Award from the Centers for Medicare and Medicaid Services in 2012 to expand the model to 13 programs in six states and Puerto Rico (now a total of 17 clinics). Data from the study, which followed patients in the network from 2012 to 2015, are being analyzed.

Moving forward, Steiner emphasized the importance of always involving multiple stakeholders and engaging communities in research, but also providing training and employment opportunities. Under a new Patient-Centered Outcomes Research Institute project called SHARE, Transitions Clinic Network will train teams of collaborators—including researchers, correctional administrators, care providers, community members, patients, and community health workers—to develop community-centric research questions and will eventually share network data with the community through a public data distribution network.

"At Transitions Clinic, we really want to ensure that our values are steeped in what the community values and needs," she said. "What's made our work most successful is that we strive to have the individual and community at the center of our collaboration."

Juvenile Prisons: Dire Health Impacts on Youth

As with the adult prison system, the picture of well-being and health care inside and outside juvenile prisons is bleak, according to a report released in February 2017. *Juvenile InJustice: Charging Youth as Adults Is Ineffective, Biased, and Harmful* examines how charging youths as adults leads to negative health impacts and how prison is detrimental to their health and well-being.[11]

According to the report, published by Health Impact Partners in partnership with the Youth Justice Coalition and Communities United for Restorative Youth Justice (CURYJ, pronounced *Courage*):

- Incarceration undermines youth health and well-being and exposes youths to higher rates of chronic and infectious disease, violence, physical abuse, and sexual abuse.

- Incarcerated youths face psychological abuse and mental health issues, including negative "identity impacts." These impacts on "development, identity formation, and life outlook may derive from incarcerated young people identifying themselves as deviant, being socialized via exposure to other incarcerated people into values considered deviant by society, and having normal elements of development such as work and family relationships disrupted."
- Juvenile incarceration is associated with negative health outcomes as an adult, including early death. Lack of rehabilitation and healing leads to high recidivism.
- Youth are 36 times more likely to commit suicide in an adult jail than in a juvenile facility.

In summary, the report noted,

> When we lock up young people, they are more likely to be exposed to extreme violence, fall prey to abuse, and suffer from illness. High rates of violence, unchecked gang activity, and overcrowding persist in Division of Juvenile Justice facilities where many youth sentenced as adults start their incarceration. Fights frequently erupt in facility dayrooms and school areas.
>
> Even if young people manage to escape direct physical abuse in juvenile or adult facilities, exposure and proximity to violence can be harmful in and of itself. Research suggests that exposure to violence can lead to issues with development in youth.

A Personal Story Connecting Criminal Justice and Well-Being

For George Galvis, the *Juvenile InJustice* report was a veritable blueprint to help explain why he has devoted his entire professional career to preventing youth from being charged as adults and to keeping them from reentering the criminal justice system. As cofounder and executive director of CURYJ, Galvis partnered with Human Impact Partners to produce the report.

Galvis had more than a professional stake in *Juvenile InJustice*. As he revealed through a story that was poignant and at times heartbreaking, this was personal. Born into a violent and abusive family of mixed Latino and American Indian heritage, Galvis's first memory growing up in the Bay Area of Northern California was of his father trying to kill his mother. He was three years old. Galvis, his sister, and his mother escaped, but they were repeatedly forced to move from address to address to avoid the man who continued to stalk and threaten them.

It took years for Galvis to understand, but "the violence that was produced in my home, I then reproduced on the streets later as a young man."

In 1992, then 17-year-old Galvis was arrested and charged with attempted murder and assault with a deadly weapon for his involvement in a drive-by shooting. Incarcerated, Galvis had what he called his "first opportunity to reflect really deeply about that." When he realized how it sounded to be the person convicted of those charges, he didn't excuse or ignore it. "Good Lord," he thought. "I sound terrible."

Charged as a youth and soon released, Galvis began what he calls "my healing journey" by working to understand his culture and his indigenous roots. Starting at a community college campus and then enrolling at the University of California, Berkeley, Galvis immersed himself in ethnic studies and comparative analysis of different racial justice movements, reading as much as he could from political and cultural sociologists, educators, and authors like Frantz Fanon, Paulo Freire, and Alfred Memmi.

For the first time in his life, Galvis said, "I had the vocabulary to articulate the things that I felt as a young person." He grew to understand that "a lot of the violence that I was consumed with during my adolescence was really me raging against my father, because I looked just like him. The men that I was engaged in conflict with looked just like me, too. It was very fratricidal in nature."

As a Ronald E. McNair Scholar and Public Policy and International Affairs Scholar, Galvis received a BA in ethnic studies and a master's in city planning from Berkeley. But Galvis didn't just pursue educational degrees. Encouraged by a janitor who befriended him at a community college, Galvis also took steps to reconnect with his culture, "taking time to feed my spirit, to help me move beyond my trauma."

Galvis emphasized that point. "I really want to punctuate that—because I don't think higher education, in itself, would have been enough. I could still be highly dysfunctional. We see this with a lot of men of color where there's still substance abuse, multiple divorces, even with doctorates, with law degrees, as social workers. Dysfunction plagues their families as a result of them not having taken that work to really heal themselves. If people don't take time to heal themselves, that trauma becomes drama. Finding my healing journey, and having a cultural outlet and being able to feed my spirit, became very instrumental in my change."

> We have an expression in Spanish, "La cultura cura"— culture is healing. And that's also true in First Nations communities. We say that culture is our strength. It's our healing and recovery.
> —George Galvis

CURYJ: Putting Personal Experiences to Work Helping Others

Two decades ago, Galvis cofounded CURYJ to promote restorative justice, cultural understanding, and healing in the violence-plagued communities of the Bay Area. As executive director and a dedicated youth activist, Galvis draws on his own experiences and indigenous roots to help young people, particularly those involved in the criminal justice system.

Galvis and his colleagues at CURYJ create programs designed to reduce youth violence while providing culturally sensitive, restorative programs to those who have been incarcerated. Galvis is partial to the phrase "hurt people, hurt people" and "healed people, heal people" and offered two examples of CURYJ programs that help heal:

- ROOTS (Reclaiming Our Original Traditions and Stories) helps Oakland's Latino and Native American youth understand the historical and contemporary manifestations of oppression by looking at their pasts. These youth are then exposed to traditional forms of healing, conflict resolution techniques, and communication skills that encourage them to be restorative justice practitioners. "Moving from a place where we have a common pain to one where we have a common struggle is one of the values that we try to operate from," said Galvis.
- In 2012, CURYJ members surveyed more than 2,000 residents across Los Angeles County about solutions to address violence. Responders could have chosen more police, more gang injunctions, or more incarceration; instead they prioritized youth centers, youth jobs, and intervention workers who strive to build peaceful relationships in schools and communities.

CURYJ also advocates for policies that positively affect at-risk youth and campaigns against legislation and policies that would have a negative impact. Two examples:

- Fundamentally opposed to gang injunctions as both ineffective and destabilizing, Galvis helped lead the Stop the Injunctions Coalition, which successfully prevented Oakland's 2010 gang injunction from being fully implemented. (Gang injunctions are civil court orders that allow police to arrest a person suspected of being a gang member by using a lower legal standard than usually required. Otherwise legal activities—for example, riding a bus with a friend—may be illegal for targeted individuals under an injunction.)

  Later, working with the young men who were defendants in a gang injunction case, Galvis helped them "move beyond that trauma and become leaders in that movement" through restorative healing techniques, political process and interdisciplinary training, and training in public speaking.

"I'm very proud to say that a number of these young men are now on my staff and are now mentors," said Galvis. "And in the city of Oakland, we are the first community-led effort in the nation—that we're aware of—to fully defeat gang injunctions. As of March 2015, the gang injunctions were lifted and all cases were dismissed."

- CURYJ has a long history of opposing Proposition 21 in California, which passed in 2001, allowing district attorneys to directly charge youth as young as 14 as adults. In 2016, Galvis and CURYJ coauthored Proposition 57, which takes away the discretion of DAs to charge youths as adults and shifts the burden of proof from the defense to the prosecution. The measure, overwhelmingly passed by voters in November 2016, was the first ballot initiative created and led largely by formerly incarcerated people and families across California.

    "Our young people, who called themselves 'Homies 4 Justice' and were too young to vote, organized a campaign called 'Get On The Bus' where they would hit the transit lines in the Bay Area [and] talk to adults, saying, 'I cannot vote, but will you be my voice?'"

The Proposition 21 issue was particularly personal for Galvis, who was tried and convicted as a juvenile when he was 17, resulting in a lesser sentence than if he had been tried as an adult. "Had I been charged in the era of Prop 21," acknowledged Galvis, "I'd probably still be incarcerated."

Reflections on Criminal Justice and Health

Lash emphasized the significance of both Transitions Clinic Network and CURYJ, saying that they are "two models of cross-sector programs that really show us how big ideas play out in the real world."

Though she acknowledged the shifting political climate and unknown budgeting changes ahead, Lash closed the session with a review of federal grant opportunities and programs that promote research and services related to criminal justice initiatives:

- The **National Criminal Justice Initiatives map**, which identifies recipients of federal funding related to reentry and recidivism reduction across the country.[12] As a joint project of the Department of Justice–funded National Reentry Resource Center and the Federal Interagency Reentry Council, this map of programs and federal investments can help policymakers, researchers, and community-based organizations identify potential partners for reentry initiatives.

- A list of **primary federal funding sources** for reentry-related research, evaluation, and projects that promote better health and employment opportunities for recently incarcerated individuals. These include grants from the National Science Foundation; the National Institute for Justice and the Bureau for Justice Assistance, both within the U.S. Department of Justice; the Employment and Training Administration, within the U.S. Department of Labor; and the Centers for Disease Control and Prevention.
- The **National Reentry Resource Center**, administered by the Department of Justice's Bureau of Justice Assistance, a goldmine of useful information and announcements about reentry programs, policies, initiatives, and grant solicitations.
- **National Clean Slate Clearinghouse**, a new program funded jointly by the Department of Justice and the Department of Labor, that recognizes the importance of civil legal assistance to help people with criminal records successfully reenter the community. The clearinghouse provides information on record clearance and mitigation, supports legal service providers currently engaged in and new to record clearance work, and gives information to policymakers to compare their state's record clearance policies to best national and regional practices.

Like Steiner and Galvis, Lash noted the importance of stakeholder collaboration and multidisciplinary research, which was highlighted in recent federal grant opportunities targeted at the criminal justice community. Prompted by questions from the audience, both Steiner and Galvis stressed the need to include formerly incarcerated individuals in all aspects of the work. Galvis often shares that message as a speaker at national events; for instance, he recently spoke about his experiencesat the national program office launch event for RWJF's *Forward Promise* program, a signature effort begun in 2012 to promote the health and well-being of boys and young men of color.

One audience member asked why exposure to violence and trauma is not recognized as a social determinant of health. The presenters reinforced that "recognizing and moving beyond violence" is now a part of their programs for incarcerated individuals. In response to another question, Steiner noted that health care providers and staff at

> *I encourage all of you to allow those who are directly impacted to be partners, not subjects, of your research. Otherwise, research is essentially recolonizing communities of color.*
> —*George Galvis*

the Transitions Clinic Network receive the same cultural humility training provided to community health workers.

There were no easy answers, however, to those who asked about the future of health care programs for formerly incarcerated individuals, especially those provided through Medicaid expansion programs under the Affordable Care Act. The criminalization of immigrants—tagged "crimmigation"—and the potential effects on well-being present another emerging issue. "This is an entirely new discussion," acknowledged Galvis, "but it's something we are mobilizing and organizing around in California."

A Final Word

With more than 2.2 million people in U.S. prisons, and many more individuals with recent experiences of incarceration, there is a vast population whose health and health care are affected by their connection with the criminal justice system. Although they live in environments with multiple sources of health risk, these individuals have limited access to timely health services, and they have little control over lifestyle and other contributors to well-being.

The conference presenters made a powerful case for the impact of involvement in the criminal justice system on health, both inside and outside prison. Taking steps to mitigate that impact will reap long-lasting benefits for a great many people, with wide-ranging positive consequences across society.

Resilience and Climate Change

BRETT KENCAIRN

Senior Climate and Sustainability Coordinator, City of Boulder

NICOLE LURIE, MD, MSPH

Former Assistant Secretary for Preparedness and Response, U.S. Department of Health and Human Services

SABRINA MCCORMICK, PHD

Associate Professor, Environmental and Occupational Health, George Washington University

ELIZABETH SAWIN, PHD

Co-director, Climate Interactive

The topic of climate change remains contentious in the United States despite the scientific consensus that it poses potentially calamitous consequences. Conference presenters acknowledged the friction, but focused their attention on the health impacts and ways to build resilience in vulnerable populations and communities disproportionately impacted by a changing planet.

A diverse panel included a filmmaker/university professor, a scientist, a city planner, and a former federal government official. In this chapter, these contributors discuss a wide range of promising strategies to empower and build resilient communities. They review "multisolving" approaches that connect climate change and health benefits, present innovative community concepts that reframe climate change for citizens, and emphasize the importance of building resilience in individuals and communities alike.

Each panel member argued that these intervention strategies will always include co-benefits for citizens' health and the environment because the two are inextricably

What can we do to empower community? With this panel, we see efforts to mitigate climate change issues and to build resilient infrastructures and communities that can respond to and even be prepared for these changing outcomes.
—Sabrina McCormick

linked. Moderator Sabrina McCormick agreed. "We cannot talk about one without the other."

A Review of the Facts

To set the stage for the session, McCormick acknowledged that in this "highly politicized environment where climate change has become a partisan issue," the evidence that climate change is real is irrefutable. "Oftentimes Americans, especially, think that climate change is a phenomenon that only affects other countries and other populations, and that's absolutely untrue," she said.

McCormick was an associate producer of *The Years of Living Dangerously,* an Emmy Award–winning documentary about climate change. "We are already seeing the effects of climate change here in the United States, and will be seeing them more and more rapidly than has even been predicted." The 2017 hurricane season, featuring Hurricanes Harvey, Irma, Maria, and others, certainly lent credence to that assertion.

McCormick reviewed the Environmental Protection Agency's definition of climate change: "Any significant change in the measure of climate lasting for an extended period of time. In other words, climate change includes major changes in temperature, precipitation, or wind patterns, among others, that last several decades or longer."

To highlight the extent of these changes, she presented a set of statistically packed graphics showing variations in the Earth's surface temperature for the past 1,000 years,[1] temperature change calculated by the Intergovernmental Panel on Climate Change since 1950 and projected into 2030, and the annual greenhouse gas index.

McCormick offered a compelling statistic: though climate variations have been documented for more than 1,000 years, a rapid incline in temperature after the Industrial Revolution has not dropped back to previous patterns of fluctuations. What's more, she said, these temperatures appear to be rising still, driven by an increase in greenhouse gas emissions like carbon dioxide, methane, and nitrous oxide.

According to the EPA, greenhouse gases trap heat and make the planet warmer, and human activities are responsible for almost all the increase in greenhouse gases in the atmosphere over the past 150 years. The largest source of greenhouse gas emissions from human activities in the United States is from burning fossil fuels for electricity, heat, and transportation.[2]

To avert what McCormick called "catastrophic climate change" consequences, she explained how the recent Paris Climate Accord proposed to take steps to lower greenhouse gas emissions and help limit rising temperatures to below 2 degrees Celsius. Without such efforts, scientists predict that temperature change in the next 100 years or so will increase 3.6 degrees, said McCormick.

McCormick pointed out that climate change is "not seasons, this is not just weather. This is not to say that we can't attribute certain proportions of extreme weather events (like hurricanes) to climate change. We can do that now." A new field of "attribution science" is helping to make that possible.

From Greenhouse Gases to "I'm Sick"

McCormick presented a schematic of different pathways that show how climate change can affect multiple health outcomes—or, as McCormick summarized, "the mechanics of how we get from those greenhouse gases to 'I'm sick.'" She listed many of the environmental and health impacts of global warming and climate change:

- **Rising sea levels and temperatures.** "We are seeing this more rapidly than we expected, with Arctic ice melt which is resulting in sea level rise globally. Half of the world's population lives on the coasts, right? So we're looking at 50 percent of the world's population at risk of sea-level rise."
- **Increased pollen production and rising reports of allergic diseases like asthma.** "Unfortunately, plants that produce pollen seem to like warmer temperatures generally, so we're going to be seeing increasing allergic diseases."
- **Rise in heat-related illnesses and deaths.** "In the United States, heat kills more people than all other extreme weather events combined. When temperature increases, it catalyzes chemical processes in the air, so we see more ground-level ozone, more exposures to people who are concerned about cardiopulmonary and respiratory diseases and asthma."
- **Coastal flooding and storm surges.** "With an increase in extreme weather–related health effects, this can be death and injury from a flood event, a hurricane, or a storm." McCormick added that in addition to drownings and injuries, these events trigger health problems associated with displaced populations that range from a lack of shelter and mold-ridden housing environments to vector- and rodent-borne diseases.
- **Drought conditions.** "When we have drought or extreme weather events, the patterns of crops change. Lack of rain can lead to decreased crop yields, and that leads to malnutrition, especially in countries and communities already living on the verge of food insecurity."
- **Proliferation of water-borne and food-borne diseases.** "The ocean is our biggest moderator of climate change—it's absorbed 80 percent of the carbon

that we've emitted so far. As the ocean warms, the seafood that we eat in the sea is also warming and so microbial contamination transmission is taking place and sometimes increasing when that temperature warms. This leads to increasing or changing patterns in water- and food-borne diseases."

- **Challenges and devastation to coastal environments that impact nature and food supplies.** "We have coastal flooding and coast aquifer salinity change, and this has a great effect, especially on protein sources for populations that are dependent on the sources of seafood in the sea."

> *There's a broad range of health effects from climate change that are occurring already around the world. We've seen them in the past decades, through extreme weather events as well as through gradual changes.*
> —Sabrina McCormick

Poking gentle fun at her dire introductory remarks and facts, McCormick stressed that she didn't want to be "the 'Debbie Downer' and tell you, 'Forget it, we're all done and there's nothing we can do.' That's absolutely the opposite of the message I want to portray."

The next three panelists, she stressed, would provide information about "the next step into empowerment" and approaches for resilience in the face of climate change.

Protecting the Environment and Improving Health

Looking around a room filled with health experts, presenter Elizabeth Sawin started with two questions: "How many of you have ever been asked by a climate or energy expert for input into the challenges they face? How many times have any of you reached out to climate and energy experts for political capital or money or support?"

Acknowledging the three or four hands raised in response to each question, Sawin did not equivocate. "We need a lot more of that. We need every hand in this room to raise. From my world of climate and energy, I don't think we're going to be able to do what needs to be done without your help. And from your world, as I hear of your visions about addressing equity and poverty and the social determinants of health, I don't think you're going to fulfill your visions if we lose on climate."

Sawin is the codirector of Climate Interactive, a not-for-profit organization in Washington that helps people understand how to address climate change and related issues like energy, water, food, and disaster risk reduction. Specifically, Climate Interactive creates interactive, scientifically rigorous simulation tools like C-ROADS and En-ROADS to illustrate connections, play out scenarios, and see what works to understand and track the impacts of climate change, clean energy, disaster risk reduction, and resilience.

Protecting the climate goes hand in hand with improving health, equity, and well-being, she said. To prove her point, Sawin referenced a 2010 study from the Health and Environmental Alliance and Health Care Without Harm called "Acting NOW for Better Health."[3] The report documented the savings in health care costs for the European Union if the EU moved its 2020 United Nations Framework Convention on Climate Change (UNFCCC) pledge to reduce greenhouse gases and emissions from 20 percent to 30 percent.

While the total costs of the program—estimated at around €45 billion over a decade—are cumulative, the health benefits are yearly and immediate. By 2020, the benefits would include 140,000 additional years of life, 13 million fewer days of restricted activity, 1.2 million fewer days of respiratory illness, 142,000 fewer consultations for upper respiratory symptoms and asthma, and 3,776 fewer hospital admissions for respiratory and cardiac conditions.

Pointing to a graph, Sawin explained that the *annual* health benefits appear to be about half of the *cumulative* cost of further reducing greenhouse emissions. "So what that says is, in one or two years, Europe would make back in the health benefits what they'd have to spend to be more ambitious on climate. Imagine how my world changed when I realized this." For a clearer analogy, Sawin compared this to how homeowners view home investments. "Imagine, if this is your own house and you invested in something and it would pay for itself in one or two or three years. We would do that. So why aren't we doing *this*? So, now I frame this question much more about, 'Why are we *not* doing it?'"

"Multisolving" Health and Environmental Issues

Sawin offered a new word to describe a broad approach to problems related to health and the environment: "multisolving"—the search for systemic solutions that help protect the climate while improving health, equity, and well-being.

To illustrate the concept of multisolving, Sawin turned to another pilot study from the United Kingdom. In 2014, Hylton Castle residents and physicians participated in a "boilers by prescription" program that provided energy-efficient upgrades to the homes of individuals suffering from chronic obstructive pulmonary diseases (COPD). Based on the fact that warmer, less damp homes have direct health benefits, new boilers, better windows, and insulation were provided to the homes of six COPD sufferers, who then reported fewer visits to the emergency room, fewer visits to their family doctor, and additional savings on energy bills in energy-efficient homes.

"So that's multisolving—from the smallest individual level all the way up to the largest national level," Sawin explained.

Big Wins Through Multisolving

Sawin pointed out that multisolving doesn't happen at scale for a number of reasons: a lack of relationships and collaborations between environmental and health experts, the tendency to view financing for these efforts in silos (spending in one department when savings accrue to another), and disparate framing of the issue (energy vs. health vs. climate vs. technology). She encouraged everyone to stay focused on what she called "the big wins"—those multisolving opportunities where there's a simultaneous gain in health and environmental benefits. She reviewed some key "big win" examples, emphasizing that each should be approached with "an eye toward equity":

- **Changing diets to more plant-based resources.** "The most emission-producing part of our food system comes from meat. And I don't have to tell you all about the health advantages of having a more plant-based diet."
- **Creating more active transportation infrastructure to promote walking and biking.** "This is obviously a big health win and it's also getting us out of our cars and reducing greenhouse gases from the transportation sector."
- **Creating more energy-efficient and healthier homes.** "As we found in the U.K., the healthier homes also had reduced energy costs, a 'big win' especially for people on low incomes."
- **Moving from dirty fossil fuel energy and creating greener urban areas to reduce air pollution and clean the air.** "Air pollution is probably the biggest health expense of our fossil fuel–dependent society. So any moves away from things like coal and diesel are a huge win for air pollution and therefore for health. And bringing green into our urban areas helps particularly with climate resilience, and you all know the health and mental health benefits of being in green space, of having nature around us."
- **Boosting social connectedness and reducing emissions by increasing sharing and reducing consumption.** "Consumption is a huge climate wedge. And there's no way to meet climate goals if we don't have lives that are embedded in communities that work and are connected."

Sawin challenged everyone at the conference to contribute to these efforts on two important levels—as private citizens with expertise that can help inform policy decisions, and as influential professionals with a say in how money will be used for environmental and health improvements. "There's going to be a huge amount of money spent in the next few decades, both getting us onto a clean energy path and helping adapt to the climate change we can't prevent," Sawin said. "But if the health community is not organized to advocate for spending that money in ways that benefit health, I think it's going to be a missed opportunity."

> *The theme can be, "All is not lost." There's actually a lot of opportunity.*
> —Elizabeth Sawin

Changing the Message

As the climate action change coordinator and senior environmental planner for Boulder, Colorado, presenter Brett KenCairn had some advice for environmental activists and health care practitioners who are worried about the climate: change the message.

"Climate change is not a problem," said KenCairn. "But we are approaching it as if it *is* a problem. Climate change, I would argue, is a symptom. Or, more accurately, it is a signal and a message from a larger living system called Earth that humans are actually not living in sustainable ways."

Responding to climate change as if it were a problem, KenCairn argued, "is just mind-boggling. Because on one day, it's about not eating meat. And another day, it's about riding the bus. And you know, it's just a mind-boggling set of 'What should I do?'"

Instead, KenCairn advocates talking about climate change in relevant and actionable ways, reframing climate issues in a positive light that emphasizes desired outcomes. For example, he suggests articulating a goal of an 80 percent increase in renewable energy (rather than an 80 percent reduction in fossil fuels). "Human behaviors move toward what they want, not away from what they don't want."

Boulder Takes Action

> *If we get our systems right—if we start to make sustainable energy systems and sustainable relationship ecosystems and use resources in a sustainable and circular way, and create sustainable relationships to each other—climate change actually takes care of itself.*
> —Brett KenCairn

KenCairn argued that the earth as a living system "is providing us very accurate and specific guidance about which of our human systems are not sustainable."

With this in mind, the city of Boulder identified and approved a new climate action plan in 2016 that mapped out actions that city's citizens could take within four distinct areas to reduce greenhouse gas emissions by 80 percent or more below 2005 levels by 2050:

- **Energy and energy systems.** Reduce fossil fuel demand from buildings and transportation. Rapidly transition to an energy system and economy that is powered 100 percent or more by renewable clean electricity with 50 percent or more of that produced locally.
- **Climate/ecosystems**. Respond to climate change in ways that create a healthier, more resilient community. Enhance the ability of urban, wildland, and agricultural ecosystems to capture and stabilize atmospheric carbon and provide critical buffering against climatic extremes.
- **Use of resources/zero waste.** Expand opportunities to reduce waste and to reuse, recycle, and compost. Reduce the emissions impacts caused by the use of goods and services by maximizing the productivity of all resources used and making purchasing decisions that support responsible resource use.
- **Social equity and community climate action.** Make all changes just and equitable to all members of the community. Support the inspiration and innovation of those who live, work, study, and visit in Boulder to create a low-carbon economy and lifestyle that improve the health, shared prosperity, and long-term security of the community.

Identifying these four areas answered KenCairn's "Where do we take action?" question. But, early in the plan's development, he realized there was a glitch: no one could smell, touch, or taste a greenhouse gas—the very thing the city's new action plan wanted to address. "So imagine, we're telling our citizens that we have to do this Herculean, civilization-changing effort to produce a whole bunch less of this thing you can't even relate to. So not such an effective branding strategy, right?"

To change the narrative, KenCairn described how the city went back to the drawing board and asked another question: "Well, what does this really mean?" KenCairn's answer broke it down into a simple answer with simple parts. The city's climate action program wanted to work with the community to understand what it would mean for Boulder to have an energy system that's 80 percent or more based on clean, renewable energy.

A traditional framing positioned climate action as a problem that had to be fixed, involving trade-offs against other municipal priorities, such as water and sewer, roads, affordable housing, public safety, and equitable social services. But under an alternative approach, climate change is not a problem but a symptom, and changes to the city's energy systems would lead to healthy affordable housing, efficient and accessible transportation, energy resilience and security, and equitable economic development.

KenCairn gave an example how a change in Boulder's energy system creates this equity transfer. He noted that Boulder spends $300 million each year on energy from fossil fuels like petroleum, natural gas, and electricity—money that essentially leaves the community. By transitioning to renewable energy, such as wind and solar power, those resources can stay in the community.

But could the city of Boulder create this future? Again, the city's climate team knew that unless the community understood how much fossil fuel energy it used and how much clean, sustainable energy it could produce, there would be no support to change that system. He called the situation a "cultural narrative problem. We have been convinced that we can't actually create this future."

To alter this perspective, the city followed the approach taken by the Solutions Project: renewable energy in every state. Using relatively simple analytic tools accessible to any community, the city was able to calculate that the community needed 350 megawatts of electric power to replace all forms of energy being used—including natural gas and petroleum. So where would they get that power?

The city's team first examined wind energy. With just 125 turbines, the city could produce the 350 megawatts of electricity needed, but it couldn't be produced locally. What about solar? How much energy falls on the rooftops in Boulder? That number turned out to be 500 megawatts on rooftops alone, which are the premium solar collectors. "That's not counting our carports, it's not our parking lots. We have one of the highest per capita solar adoption rates in this country—20 MW of installed solar. However, this meant we needed to look for strategies to increase this by nearly 20 times."

The ultimate take-away, KenCairn said, "is that now our community knows we can get there. We have shown our community how we can create an energy system in which probably 75 percent of that money stays in our community. And if we developed our incentives right, that money would be staying in the pockets of a lot of the families that need it most. That's a part of the multisolving opportunities that we have with this. A better energy system could actually lower living costs and improve air quality."

By changing the narrative of climate change and selling the public on the co-benefits of taking action, KenCairn believes strongly that citizens will buy in. "People aren't going to spend the money that they have to spend because it's going to somehow save the planet. I'm sorry—but I'm going to tell you that right now. People aren't going to make those decisions unless they see personal benefit."

There are some hopeful signs out there. It's really a set of choices that we need to offer our community about where we want to go.
—Brett KenCairn

Stories of Resilience Through Disasters

For eight years, Nicole Lurie served as assistant secretary for preparedness and response in the U.S. Department of Health and Human Services. The office was created in 2006 under the Pandemic and All Hazards Preparedness Act in the wake of Hurricane Katrina to lead the nation in preventing, preparing for, and responding to the adverse health effects of public health emergencies and disasters.

That work allowed Lurie to study how different kinds of disasters— particularly ones related to extreme weather or disease outbreaks—can build resilience in the long run. "Numerous events have taught us about building resilience," she said, pointing to a timeline of disasters from 2001 to 2016 that included 9/11, anthrax attacks, Hurricanes Katrina and Rita, the Haiti earthquake, outbreaks of H5N1 influenza (so-called bird flu), the Sandy Hook shooting and the Boston Marathon bombing, the Zika virus, and the Flint, Michigan, water crisis, to name but a few. (And, of course, her presentation preceded the catalog of devastating storms and fires in 2017.)

"Never let a good disaster go to waste," she suggested. "We always have to learn from it, and do better."

Circles of Impact

Lurie explained how her work was guided by a National Health Security Strategy, adopted in 2010, which focuses not only on emergency management systems and emergency responses but on building community resilience, strengthening situational awareness to support decision-making, and integrating health, health care, and emergency management systems. "It really posits that individuals and communities that are more resilient do better and bounce back better in the face of disasters," she said.

> *Most people judge how bad something was by how quickly they recover.*
> —*Nicole Lurie*

Lurie described the "circles of impact" that climate change and environmental disasters have on the physical and mental health of communities. After natural disasters, people often suffer from stress, anxiety, depression, grief, and a sense of loss; strained social and personal relationships; higher levels of substance abuse; and posttraumatic stress disorders. Too, she noted that community health is impacted in adverse ways, ranging from an increase in interpersonal aggression, violence, and crime to decreases in social stability and community cohesion.

"Psychological impacts are one of the most important and overlooked aspects of resilience," she noted. She illustrated the concept of organizational resilience with a picture of the Japanese women's soccer team after it won the Women's World Cup, right after the Fukushima earthquake in 2011. "If there's one thing I take away from all the work that's been done on resilience over the past decade, it's really about this issue—about social capital and funding and bridging social capital. Organizational resilience on any level is just really, really important."

Building Resilience After Bad Things Happen

Lurie shared examples of how federal agencies and communities learn from disasters to help build strategies for resilience.

- **Emergency preparedness.** After Hurricane Katrina and Superstorm Sandy, hospitals, clinics, dialysis centers, and other health care systems had points of failure that adversely impacted not only patient care but employee safety. Today, as a condition of participation in Medicare, the Centers for Medicare and Medicaid Services requires all health care institutions to establish and be able to execute emergency preparedness plans. These plans must address:
  - Physical infrastructure, electronic health records, responses to different scenarios such as hurricanes, floods, fires, epidemic outbreaks.
  - Health care coalitions that will work together when segments of a hospital and clinic system fail in order to accommodate all patients during a disaster.
  - Systems that are prepared for highly infectious diseases, especially during epidemics of fear.
  - Behavioral health plans that are integrated into the rest of health care planning. "One of the most important things that we did was start to integrate behavior health," said Lurie. "Think about it: if you lose your home, your livelihood, if it takes two years to get your home fixed up and rebuilt, you're suffering a lot on a lot of different levels. It keeps you and your family from functioning in a lot of different ways. We need a really different approach to this and a much more population approach to all of that."
- **Emerging disease outbreaks and countermeasure responses.** Lessons from each outbreak have helped the United States build a capable medical countermeasure response infrastructure that includes vaccines and treatment.
  - Capabilities built after the H1N1 epidemic in 2009 were later leveraged for Ebola and Zika responses.

- The Coalition for Epidemic Preparedness Innovation, launched in 2016, formed to provide a global perspective on preparedness for existing disease outbreaks and to produce vaccines quickly when new diseases emerge.
- **Data to support a population approach to resilience and help support equity.** "I think we all know that, in general, populations that are poor, less educated, often nonwhite in this country suffer much more from disasters because they live in more disaster-prone areas," said Lurie. "It's possible to use really basic data—again, this isn't rocket science—to create a population-based approach to identify populations in need and living most on the edge, and think about interventions that you can put in place to help them."

  Lurie noted that this system was used to identify pockets of Vietnamese-speaking communities after the Gulf Coast oil spill and to identify communities hit hardest by a recent drought in the Midwest.
- **Preparing for electrical failures and prescription drug shortages.** When the electricity goes out, millions of people around the country who live on electrically dependent medical equipment are at risk. Frustrated that they could not be identified quickly, Lurie worked through her agency to create a new system called Empower that stores the addresses of people with electrical medical equipment, encourages local planners to anticipate their needs, and moves quickly to help them in emergencies. "You can never tell me again that you didn't know those people lived in the community," said Lurie.

  Another lesson is that people run out of medicine following disasters. Through partnerships with major drugstores, refill alerts are now sent via text or email to remind people to refill prescriptions when a major storm is predicted. Likewise, after dialysis patients in New Orleans became ill or died after Hurricane Katrina, an alert system was set up before Superstorm Sandy, allowing dialysis to be scheduled in advance—"preventive dialysis, in a sense," said Lurie. "We were able to show that you reduced adverse outcomes, reduced emergency department visits, hospitalizations, or deaths. And now we have data for a quality measure of best practice."
- **Recognizing the psychological impacts of environmental degradation.** The psychological impacts of "environmental degradation and fear make people sick," said Lurie, citing two specific behavioral health concerns: (1) an epidemic of fear caused by excessively prevalent and contagious perception of dangers and (2) "solastalgia," a term coined in 2003 and defined as "the anguish felt when one's home environment is damaged or degraded."

  Pointing out that building health resilience builds psychological resilience, Lurie called for incorporating behavioral health considerations and social connectedness into disaster preparedness plans. Groups like Team Rubicon during the Louisiana flooding, Islamic Relief USA in Louisiana and North

Carolina, and youth groups engaged in response and recovery are examples of using connectedness to build resiliency.

Looking around the conference room, Lurie concluded with a call to action: "We can't get better unless we study this. We need, as a research community and a public health community, to figure out how we do the kind of research to build resilience before climate-related disasters happen, and during and after those events."

Reflections on a Changing Planet

Following the discussion, McCormick observed that the panelists had integrated "the way we think about climate change with thinking about health, and seeing how we can't really think about one without the other. And we're talking about the transformation of systems that have the potential to really affect the way our societies work."

Concerns were raised, however, about how those systems could establish equity for all citizens. One audience member, for instance, asked how indigenous populations could be protected from economic developments that destroy their environments, with examples ranging from the Amazon rainforest deforestation projects to U.S. pipeline construction efforts that threaten communities like Standing Rock.

The question brought a range of responses. Sawin reminded everyone that "indigenous peoples are responsible for much of the remaining forest capacity on the planet, so their role as stewards is a really important lever that we shouldn't forget." And KenCairn allowed that we need better relationships with native communities, in part because they have a lot to teach about "disruptive change. That's what resilience is all about—how do we relate to disruptive change? Indigenous societies have always understood that."

Other questions from the audience zeroed in on local activism in an issue as obviously global as climate change. Michael W. Painter, JD, MD, senior program officer with the Robert Wood Johnson Foundation, pointed out that so much about building a Culture of Health vision "devolves down to a local level, and people doing things in their community. But when you think about climate change, it is this planetary issue that we, as a global community, have to come together and do something about. But there's also this local theme. How important is local activism in the overall effort to address climate change?"

All three panelists swiftly responded that local efforts are critical. "That's where people live, work, vote, [and] organize. It's got to happen at the local level," said Lurie. KenCairn said he believes that cities are where "the cutting edge of this work is going to happen." And Sawin responded that she has shifted her professional focus from working at the United Nations to working with watersheds within cities. "So my personal bet is on the local," she said. "Partly, that's because of this silo issue that I named; you get high enough in governments and the branches don't talk to each other. But in a neighborhood, when you talk about water and health and people and jobs, it's all the same people. So that's where I see a lot of hope."

As the contributors so cogently argued, attention to climate change must be part of any serious effort to improve health, address economic and social determinants that influence it, and reduce health inequalities. Building resilience and multisolving are big-picture approaches to tackling the effects of a changing climate and first steps in allowing local and national efforts to meet the challenges ahead.

Climate change will no doubt continue to be a divisive issue in the United States. Ongoing changes in policy and practice, and the sequence of destructive natural disasters and subsequent recovery efforts in the months after the *Sharing Knowledge* conference have continued to stimulate public discourse.

Making the Economic Case for Population Health

CATHERINE ANDERSON, MPA

Senior Vice President, Policy and Strategy, United Healthcare Community & State

DARRELL J. GASKIN, PHD, MS

Associate Professor of Health Economics; Deputy Director, Center for Health Disparities Solutions, Bloomberg School of Public Health, Johns Hopkins University

DARSHAK SANGHAVI, MD

Chief Medical Officer and Senior Vice President of Translation, OptumLabs

NIRAV R. SHAH, MD, MPH

Senior Vice President and Chief Operating Officer for Clinical Operations, Kaiser Permanente Southern California

NIRAV SHAH, MPA

Director, Social Investment Team, Social Finance

Social injustice comes with a hefty price tag. It's not cost-less to do nothing.
—*Darrell J. Gaskin*

Disparities in health based on race, ethnicity, and income have economic consequences for communities, states, and the country, in addition to the consequences for physical and mental well-being that are well-documented in this volume. "If you won't listen to the preacher, maybe you'll listen to the statesman," urges Darrell J. Gaskin, putting a poetic spin on the argument for taking action and meaning that if the moral and compassionate case for addressing disparities is not enough, the economic case should be considered as well. Likewise, an economic argument can be made for investing in prevention strategies to influence long-term health outcomes.

Many policymakers, practitioners, and funders support substantial, long-term investments in health, at least philosophically. But such efforts can be expensive and the return on the initial investment may not be evident for many years. Moreover, insurance markets have a significant amount of turnover as individuals move from one plan to another, perhaps in and out of Medicaid and, at some point, to Medicare. As a result, the benefits of reducing medical costs for a healthier population may accrue to entities that did not make the initial investment—the well-known "wrong pocket" problem.

Other characteristics of the American health care system also have important financial implications. Good health is dependent on appropriate and coordinated social supports (e.g., food security, safe housing, and accessible transportation) that are often lacking in the disadvantaged communities least able to absorb the economic burden of an unhealthy population. This burden is made especially heavy by fragmented health and social services that impact both the efficiency of care and health outcomes. In addition, evidence-based interventions, which can offer good economic value, are not considered often enough, nor is the reality that cost savings from health improvement efforts may be offset by the costs of increased longevity. An encouraging development is the emergence of innovative funding strategies that bring increased financial resources to the system.

The contributors to this chapter address all of this and more as they explore the economics of tackling health care disparities, social determinants of health, and other influences on health outcomes. Their conclusion is clear: investing to improve wellness and health among all people pays off.

The Cost of Health Disparities

Addressing health disparities is not only the right thing to do, said Gaskin, but "it is also the most sensible thing to do. If you don't do anything it still is going to cost you money." Gaskin and colleagues at George Washington University and Uniform Services University of the Health Sciences conducted two studies that support this view.

In research conducted by the Joint Center for Political and Economic Studies, investigators identified the direct costs of providing health care to a population that is sicker and more disadvantaged as a result of disparities as well as the indirect costs of lost productivity and wages, absenteeism, family leave, and early death.[1]

Over a four-year period (2003–06), the total costs associated with health disparities in the United States totaled $1.24 trillion, of which $229.4 billion was spent on direct medical care expenditures for people of color. During this period, 30.6 percent of direct medical care expenditures for African-American, Asian, and Hispanic people in the United States were caused by health inequalities.

A study for the Urban League focused on health care costs and lost productivity.[2] The researchers found that health disparities cost the U.S. economy $82.2 billion in 2009, including increased health care spending of $59.9 billion. African Americans accounted for $45.3 billion of that burden. While these extra costs are a significant burden to Medicaid and Medicare, they are shared by all payers. Together, private health insurers and individuals (through out-of-pocket payments) actually pay more: 38 and 28 percent, respectively. Health care costs associated with health inequities are comparable to those of serious diseases such as heart disease, cancer, and mental illness.

Labor market productivity was reduced by $22.3 billion, with a $9.8 billion loss to Hispanic people, just ahead of African Americans at $9.6 billion. The impact of lost productivity is felt across all industries—from education, health, and social services to manufacturing, professional services, construction, and elsewhere.

Groups in Michigan[3] and Texas[4] are seeking to motivate state policymakers to address health disparities. By breaking down the cost of health disparities in these states, researchers hope to bolster the case for paying attention to this issue. "Everyone should be invested in trying to address this problem," said Gaskin.

Strategies Aimed at Return on Investment

Darshak Sanghavi was previously director of Preventive and Population Health at the Center for Medicare and Medicaid Innovation (CMMI). He offered three examples of CMMI strategies for addressing issues related to return on investments in long-term population health.

Create a Surrogate Endpoint

Heart disease is the leading killer of people in the Medicare population, and many major cardiac problems can be avoided by appropriate prevention services. Previous pay-for-performance programs have focused on targets such as blood pressure or cholesterol level—"blunt instruments," as Sanghavi called them.

The Million Hearts Cardiovascular Risk Reduction model relies on a calculator developed by the American College of Cardiology and the American Heart Association to show 10-year risk of heart attack or stroke based on a variety of inputs in an algorithm with good reliability. Through bonus payments, the model creates an incentive for providers to drive down this 10-year risk for their Medicare patients, encouraging them to treat high-risk patients appropriately and not overtreat those at low risk.

"The idea was to create an intermediate, meaningful risk score that could be updated yearly," said Sanghavi. "This is how we solved the long-term outcome problem."

"Atomize" Interventions

With this strategy, CMMI sought to "atomize" investments in social determinants of health and created three tracks to test specific components:

- **Track 1, Awareness:** Screen beneficiaries to identify unmet health-related social needs and refer them to available community services.
- **Track 2, Assistance:** In addition to screening and referral, provide navigation services to help beneficiaries obtain community services and test the effectiveness of referral and navigation on total cost of care through rigorous evaluation.
- **Track 3, Alignment:** Make community-level investments that encourage partnered efforts to ensure the availability and responsiveness of community services.

CMMI assigned a dollar value to each service and used economic modeling to project the impact on the total cost of care in the Medicare population.

Change the Rules

The Diabetes Prevention Program, presented in collaboration with the YMCA, is a lifestyle intervention designed to improve the health status of people with diabetes. More than 15 years of data have demonstrated that the program reduces the risk of progression of type 2 diabetes, according to Sanghavi.

CMMI researchers were interested in the long-term value of the program and extended the period in which to measure cost savings from one or two years, which is fairly typical, to a 10- to 15-year timeline. "That was the first time that a modeling exercise had been done in an innovation-based model," noted Sanghavi.

While the program showed a $500 savings in the cost of care for a person's first quarter of participation, CMMI actuaries would not certify the program as having long-term savings. The problem? The model showed that program participants lived longer than nonparticipants, resulting in higher costs.

CMMI staff solved that by writing a new policy that acknowledged beneficiaries may have greater longevity because disease progression is prevented and outcomes improved. The policy stated, "The Centers for

Medicare and Medicaid Services made a determination that costs associated with expected improvements in longevity are not appropriate for consideration in the evaluation of program spending." The policy was approved and now holds.

An audience member asked how health and societal benefits can be balanced with the need to recognize the real costs associated with living longer as a result of prevention efforts. While the actuarially sound approach may be to zero out extended life, Sanghavi asserts that critical ethical principles need to be embedded in how we use data. "Seeing longer life as a net cost actually embodies a very specific ethos of what we think about prevention. I felt that's not who we are as Americans. That was the way we made that argument."

A Local Approach

Motivated partly by a social justice argument and partly by an economic burden argument, the state of Maryland created Health Enterprise Zones (HEZs). These are economically disadvantaged communities, or clusters of contiguous communities, that have demonstrated poor health outcomes, such as lower life expectancy or higher percentage of low-birthweight infants.

HEZs are supported in Baltimore, Annapolis, two communities in rural areas, and one in the suburbs, and have the goals of

- Reducing health disparities among racial and ethnic groups within the zones
- Improving health care access and health outcomes in underserved communities
- Reducing health care costs and hospital admissions and readmissions

While these communities have common health problems, their underlying causes differ, as do the types of available community-based resources and how they approach long-term sustainability. "One of the beauties" of HEZs, said Gaskin, is the flexibility with which they can tackle issues. The state provides each HEZ with tools to address disparities and then holds the HEZ accountable for measureable health and health care outcomes. Incentives include tax credits, loan repayment, and technical support.

The HEZs have different signature projects depending on community needs. For example, one county may need transportation because it is so dispersed while another has substance abuse and mental health needs that it wants to address through a mobile mental health van. The Baltimore site doesn't need physicians, but it does need care managers to work in the community.

From 2013 to 2016, Maryland invested more than $16.4 million in the five HEZs. An economic analysis by Johns Hopkins researchers found they had a substantial economic impact on the state:

- Over the four years, the initiative stimulated $22 million in gross outputs, $5.6 million in earnings, and 183.3 jobs per million dollars of funding.
- While emergency department use increased in HEZs, relative to HEZ-eligible communities that had not been awarded an HEZ, hospital discharges decreased substantially during the program's first three years. The net savings were about $210 million in hospital charges avoided (in Maryland, charges are tied to actual costs).

Policymakers who want to do the right thing can be put off by a program's cost, said Gaskin, "so we want to show them that doing the right thing can be cost saving."

Addressing Social Determinants of Health: Economic Necessity

Other examples of building the economic case for addressing social determinants of health come from two health care systems, one for profit, the other a nonprofit.

UnitedHealthcare: Tackling Social Needs

UnitedHealthcare Community & State, a component of the health benefits company, serves individuals who are economically disadvantaged, medically underserved, or have disabilities and complex health care needs. It participates in Medicaid, the Children's Health Insurance Program, and other federal and state health care programs that serve these populations. With more than 6 million members in 26 states, "this puts us squarely in the crosshairs of looking at how to address social needs and the economic realities of doing so," said Catherine Anderson of UnitedHealthcare.

An average of 40 percent of health care costs are driven by social and economic factors, with as much as 70 percent in some populations, said Anderson. While individual and community needs differ, disconnected social supports affect all parties in the health care system and can undermine efforts at prevention.

Inevitably, preventive care is going to be lower on the priority list of a mother worried about feeding her children. Providers can't readily help patients manage their diabetes if they lack access to healthy food or refrigeration for their insulin. Community-based organizations can't deliver effective services to people with unmanaged medical conditions. All of this affects health plans, which face poor quality ratings when their patient populations do not get the care they need.

But efforts to put together a package of needed services face many challenges. Providers often do not have access to the social data that would help them understand an individual's broader circumstances. While it is possible to use an ICD-10 code to flag homelessness and other social needs, that option is greatly underutilized.

UnitedHealthcare includes information about the codes in its provider education strategy because some providers don't even know they are available, while others need help to learn how to ask patients relevant questions, according to Anderson. Providers are offered financial incentives to question patients and increase their use of the codes.

A further challenge is that community services are often fragmented and difficult to coordinate, with different eligibility requirements that force individuals to go to multiple places to receive services. That has prompted UnitedHealthcare to focus on system integration. "We have lives we are responsible for, we have financial motivation and incentives to do so, and states are encouraging it through competitive design," said Anderson. The company supports initiatives that serve more than its own membership as it begins to address community outcomes.

A Focus on Housing

From a social perspective, perhaps the most significant issue faced by UnitedHealthcare members is housing. The organization has built relationships with the supportive housing community, matched U.S. Department of Housing and Urban Development (HUD) data with its own health care data to identify needs, and looked for ways to coordinate with relevant agencies and organizations. Using tax credits, the company has invested more than $300 million in the community to improve housing opportunities. As well, given that many states allow investments from an insurer's reserve capital, UnitedHealthcare is looking at opportunities to direct its reserve to further increase housing stock.

> *We have been somewhat forced into addressing social determinants because there is no other option for us.*
> —Catherine Anderson

UnitedHealthcare Accountable Health Communities: Hawaii

UnitedHealthcare has been awarded a Track 3 Accountable Health Communities grant from the CMMI to help mitigate severe homelessness on the Hawaiian island of Oahu, where housing is exceptionally costly. About 500 United members have an ICD-10 homeless code, and there are likely many more who are not coded.

Homeless members have a 400 percent medical loss ratio (the proportion of premium revenues spent on clinical services and quality improvement), so an intervention is clearly in the insurer's interest. "We are working closely with this state to address not only our members' needs, but, if we're successful, the needs of all of this geographic area," Anderson explained.

Sharing Data

Community-based organizations, providers, and states need data to help identify the range and depth of social needs. UnitedHealthcare has developed a series of dashboards that can help answer questions like: What is the reality of social needs? What is the impact on health care of individuals with a social need? The goal is to help those who are trying to align services and make investments. "As our data become more sophisticated, we can be far more impactful on the policy conversation," Anderson noted.

Solutions to Address Individual and Community Needs: myConnections

A set of services under the myConnections umbrella addresses the needs not only of UnitedHealthcare members, but of individuals throughout the community.

- myMoney Connect targets people who lack banking relationships, providing access to opportunities to learn how to use a bank, obtain a debit card, upload a paycheck, manage an account, and develop financial literacy.
- myData Connection is a suite of solutions that coordinates data to use as both a referral tool and as a tracking mechanism to determine the impact of referrals.
- Other solutions include myCommunity Connect, myHousing Connect, myRide connect, and myWork connect.

Because the health plan does not have access to health care spending data for nonmembers, who represent the large majority of those impacted, determining program effectiveness is often difficult. To overcome that challenge,

UnitedHealthcare is studying the impact of small pilot interventions that can be tracked with focused datasets.

For example, the company is tracking the medical spending of people with diabetes or prediabetes after a mobile food market was established in Raleigh, North Carolina, to make fresh food and resources about cooking available in their communities and to improve health outcomes. After six months, 62 percent of participants reported that their health was good or very good, compared with only 20 percent when the program started.

Kaiser Permanente: Making the Business Case

Former New York State Health Commissioner Nirav R. Shah joined Kaiser Permanente Southern California in 2014 and began to explore the business case for addressing social determinants of health among Kaiser Permanente's members. "The easiest place to look," he said, "is our most expensive members."

At Kaiser Permanente, 1 percent of members are responsible for 29 percent of spending.[5] On average in 2015, Kaiser Permanente spent $98,000 for each of these members versus an average of $2,500 for everyone else. These individuals have multiple chronic conditions, including diabetes, mental illness, and asthma, among others. While some are homeless or dual eligible (receiving both Medicaid and Medicare), 22 percent are commercial members.

Despite this extraordinary level of spending, Nirav R. Shah does not believe that Kaiser Permanente is meeting the total health needs of the highest cost patients. "We do well with medium-risk patients," he said—those with just diabetes or just hypertension. But for those at highest risk, with multiple chronic conditions, "the model breaks down," he admitted. "We could all do better for these individuals."

So what to do?

In conjunction with Health Leads, which connects patients with community-based organizations to meet their social needs, Kaiser Permanente conducted a randomized trial of 5,000 high-risk members.[6] Of 2,500 who agreed to be screened, 52 percent identified one or more social needs, with an average of 3.5 unmet social needs apiece. Those most often mentioned were related to finances, caregiver support, and food. Ultimately 483 high-risk individuals were connected with community-based services. "This is not us solving their problems," Nirav R. Shah pointed out. "We just identified the need and connected the individual to housing, to food, etc."

Examples of the social-needs screening questions and the percentage of respondents answering "yes" are as follows[7]:

- Within the past 12 months, have you been unable to afford to eat balanced or healthy meals? (35 percent)
- Within the past 12 months, have you thought, "The food I bought just didn't last, and I didn't have enough money to get more?" (32 percent)
- Do you have difficulty arranging for transportation to or from your medical appointments? (26 percent)
- Do you need help finding ways to pay your utility bills? (23 percent)
- Do you worry about having a safe place to live or being homeless? (13 percent)
- In the past month, have you had concerns about the conditions or quality of your housing? (13 percent)

Nirav R. Shah and the team have also found that 10 percent of community resources provide approximately 90 percent of the benefit to members. Startlingly, they also found that some 27 percent of community resources actually *hurt* members rather than help them. Kaiser Permanente will assist some of these organizations with performance improvement training, although Shah acknowledges that "some of them probably need to be shut down."

> *We can make the business case. We can't afford not to do it. And it's our mission and the right thing to do.*
> *—Nirav R. Shah*

The experience of the large clinical trial will inform Kaiser Permanente's understanding and management of the total cost of care for all its members. "Our goal is to curate—not just for the 1 percent but for all of our members—the social, nonmedical space," explained Shah. His intent is to ensure that Kaiser Permanente decides how to spend its community benefit dollars on the basis of data and evidence.

Leveraging Resources to Promote Evidence-Based Impact

Social Finance, a nonprofit organization dedicated to mobilizing capital to drive social progress through Pay for Success, is pursuing still another economically sustainable strategy to improve population health. The organization seeks out "evidence-based programs that are measurably improving lives," said Nirav Shah, director at Social Finance (no relation to Nirav R. Shah), and works to scale those organizations to spread the benefit further. Pay for Success bonds, also called *social impact bonds*, is a funding model that combines nonprofit expertise, private sector funding, and rigorous measurement and evaluation to transform how government leaders respond to chronic social issues.

The goal of Pay for Success is to improve the lives of people in need by directing government resources toward effective programs. It sits at the intersection of three important movements:

- **Focusing on what works.** Nirav Shah noted that, of $800 billion spent annually on social services, only about 1 percent is grounded in evidence-based interventions.[8] "We need to shift that narrative and focus on the outcomes."
- **Government accountability.** "How do we ensure that we're using data, measurement, and evaluation to understand what is actually happening with taxpayer dollars?" Social Finance helps governments and investors focus their funding on programs that achieve measurable outcomes for participants. By supporting governments in utilizing data to inform decision-making, linking payments to performance, and actively managing provider operations, their work puts accountability and impact front and center.
- **Impact investing,** "using private capital as an engine to produce social good."

How Does Pay for Success Work?

Three main stakeholders are involved in Pay for Success financing: an outcomes payer, typically a government; impact investors; and one or more social service providers. A Pay for Success project specifies the outcomes of interest, how outcomes will be measured to define success, and payment terms (conditions triggering payments).

The process works like this:

- Government identifies the social need that it seeks to address.
- Social Finance raises upfront, private capital that is motivated to achieve tangible social outcomes while also generating financial returns.
- That capital is used to expand services of a nonprofit service provider to measurably and meaningfully improve outcomes to address the need government wants to tackle.
- This long-term capital (typically four to seven years) enables nonprofits to reach more individuals with programs that have been shown to deliver outcomes.
- The nonprofits serve their target population with an evidence-based intervention.
- If the program measurably improves the lives of participants, according to the specified outcomes, government repays investors.
- If no outcomes are achieved, government does not pay investors.

"The goal here is to use government, which in many circumstances is the most efficient capital, to actually scale programming to reach the broadest number of individuals," Nirav Shah said. The triple aim? "Have better population outcomes, improve quality and care, and bend the cost curve."

Government can't easily spend money for upstream investments, so this approach "allows private investors to come in on the front end," Nirav Shah explained. Operating without the regulations of Medicaid and Medicare, private capital can focus on social determinants of health, which are not generally addressed by current health care payer systems.

Nurse–Family Partnership in South Carolina: A Pay for Success Example

Nurse–Family Partnership pairs nurses with first-time, low-income mothers to support healthy pregnancies, help mothers become knowledgeable and responsible parents, and give their babies the best possible start in life. Multiple randomized controlled trials over three decades have provided strong evidence for its effectiveness.

The South Carolina Pay for Success Project is scaling Nurse–Family Partnership statewide to reach 3,200 additional mothers and their children by mobilizing $30 million. The Pay for Success financing vehicle made sense for several reasons:

- Scaling requires significant upfront investment in nonprofit infrastructure, which is difficult for Medicaid to do. Private capital provides up-front funding directed toward outcome-oriented programs that allow nonprofits to scale.
- South Carolina's Department of Health and Human Services wanted to provide access to evidence-based services for hard-to-reach, rural communities and test results there.
- South Carolina wanted to use Pay for Success to build a pathway for Medicaid to fund Nurse–Family Partnership services.
- A randomized controlled trial is being conducted to evaluate the impact of a low-cost Nurse–Family Partnership model.

Under a 1915B waiver, Medicaid provided $13 million on a reimbursement basis and Social Finance raised $17 million in private capital. This "braided capital" has enabled the project to move forward. If it achieves positive outcomes, the project will allow the South Carolina Department of Health and Human Services to use Medicaid to cover a greater percentage of Nurse–Family Partnership costs.

Outcomes are being measured through a six-year randomized controlled trial and include reduction in preterm births, improvement in healthy birth intervals, reduction in emergency department utilization in the child's first year, and assessment of the program's ability to enroll 65 percent of mothers from zip codes with the highest concentration of poverty.

This use of "private capital braided with Medicaid dollars allows a mechanism to build sustainability such that government can pick up the tab if positive outcomes are achieved," said Nirav Shah. He also mentioned work under way in Fresno and Baltimore (home remediation to mitigate children's asthma-related emergency department use and hospitalization) and Connecticut (family stability and substance use disorders).

Putting Pay for Success Into Practice

Interest in Pay for Success was high among audience members, who asked a number of questions about some of its features.

Government Buy-In

Audience question: Does government involvement in Pay for Success programs depend on whether Medicare and Medicaid participate, or do other parts of the government also have a role to play?

Experience from Social Finance has indicated that there are "pockets of opportunities in leadership" at the state level, said Nirav Shah. New York, for example, is willing to finance a prevention initiative through Pay for Success because it sees long-term benefits, especially in managed care settings where benefits can be built into capitation rates. Some states are not willing to become involved without federal assistance, however.

Participation Without Large Government Support

Audience question: When an initiative does not have large government support and someone willing to absorb costs that are not completely their own, is there hope?

Government pickup of these programs is increasing, said Nirav Shah, who is seeing more willingness to consider social benefits alongside financial benefits. "Governments are starting to build in the concept of social value," he said. There is more of a focus on the ratio of dollars spent to impact created, with governments considering how to improve the lives of their constituents, and create more equal opportunity.

Balancing Financial Savings and Moral Obligation

Audience question: Two visions are at play with regard to policies directed at social determinants of health: a legal/moral obligation and the right financing mechanism to bolster the ratio of impact and dollars spent. How can these be balanced with regard to social needs?

Social Finance's goal is to "see if there's overlap between those two dynamics of better health and better fiscal spending all in one," said Nirav Shah. If there is no overlap, this mechanism doesn't work, but there are lots of opportunities when there is.

Reflections on Policy and Practice

Other aspects of the economic case for addressing population health also prompted thoughts and questions from conference attendees.

Leveraging Medicaid Payment Reform

Audience question: Might Medicaid payment reform efforts be directed at social determinants and disparities—and what would the limitations be? Can these ideas exist in fee-for-service environments, or are they more likely to be advanced by alternative payment models?

Nirav R. Shah noted that there are models from many states and cited examples from his experience as New York State health commissioner:

- Medicaid paid for water fluoridation, recognizing that a dollar spent on fluoridation saved Medicaid $14 in children's dental bills.
- Putting $388 million of state-only funds into supportive housing saved $1 billion in care for people who would otherwise be in nursing homes and for homeless people revolving through emergency rooms.

Shah suggested collecting these kinds of ideas so that they would be available for states with block grants to use as "ideas off the shelf that the feds have already approved."

Anderson acknowledged the flexibility that comes from being outside the Medicaid fee-for-service environment. But she expressed concern with using Medicaid to cover social needs since the costs of such investments (e.g., housing) generally continue well after the medical cost savings have been realized. She suggested that a broader conversation was needed about how best to provide the range of supports that Medicaid recipients often need.

Persuading Agencies to Use Evidence-Based Interventions

Audience question: How can state Medicaid agencies be encouraged to take on interventions that have shown strong evidence of cost savings when they are not convinced they will work for their population?

In Sanghavi's view, some Medicaid agencies may have nonfinancial reasons for not offering an intervention. "You try to understand why people are not doing what you think might be necessary and then you try to work with them, either through persuasion and data and, if not, then through your political capital."

Connecting Communities and Systems

Audience question: What are ways to connect community organizations to further system integration?

UnitedHealthcare looks for "strategic partnerships with organizations that are already meeting a need," said Anderson, focusing on what it can bring to the table, such as direct financial investment or data to further decision-making. Similarly, Kaiser Permanente's goal, said Nirav R. Shah, is to build bridges to existing organizations, not to build new organizations—being careful not to overwhelm partners with its 4 million members.

Gaskin stressed the importance of building relationships by providing settings for different organizations to talk with one another and share data and information.

Life Expectancy as an Equity Issue

Audience question: Recognizing life expectancy as an equity issue, how can the United States do better?

"The idea that we as a country believe everyone should have a right to the same life expectancy [controlling for genetic differences] is worth putting a stake in the ground for," said Soma Stout, MD, from 100 Million Healthier Lives. She pointed out that similar countries "do a much better job at the same or lower cost in managing life expectancy and social well-being by coordinating in a more seamless way and removing duplication."

Sanghavi offered several levers: "(1) appeal to people's higher angels, (2) make it worth their money, and (3) regulate them and force them to play better together."

Several states, Anderson said, are considering pilots to reduce inefficiency and address community or individual needs in a different way. The challenge is identifying the path forward and overcoming the barriers. Effective partnerships are key since states and the federal government are linked in many programs.

Spending on Social Services Versus Health Care

Audience question: Is it politically feasible to allocate more resources to social services if it means shrinking health care spending?

European countries spend about 10 to 11 percent of gross domestic product (GDP) on health care and about 13 to 14 percent on social services, while the United States spends 17 percent of GDP on health care and only about 6 to 7 percent on social services, according to an audience member from Rand Corporation. The combined total percentage in each case is roughly the same; it is the allocation that differs.

Anderson pointed out that "the reality is that in health care we're spending money on social services." While there would likely be a reduction in health care spending over time, "we are already diverting health care dollars for other things today."

"Health is not the only policy," Gaskin stressed. He noted that important outcomes in education and in housing are being neglected. "Society is going to have to think about how to change this funding system so that more societal resources are in the areas in which we need to have them."

A Final Word

The Robert Wood Johnson Foundation's Culture of Health Action Framework emphasizes "making health a shared value" as one of four Action Areas. By giving due consideration to the interweaving of economic and health benefits that result from thoughtful and creative investment, the initiatives described in this chapter illuminate ways in which complex views and expectations about the value of health play out for individuals, communities, businesses, and the nation as a whole.

The economic case is clear: health disparities diminish the value of health and cost money. The sizable outlay of resources required to tackle them is readily justified both by the measurable benefits to health and well-being and the long-term economic gains. Recognizing this, many governments and organizations are stepping up to the plate to act. The time is now for others to follow their lead.

THE POWER
OF COLLABORATIVE
RELATIONSHIPS

Creating and sustaining health equity across all communities and building a Culture of Health requires that we weave an intricate web of ties across fields and disciplines. The process must be transparent, and it is inevitably complex and layered as well. Although shared interests and countless intersections provide the incentive to collaborate, effective relationships also call on us to meld very different worldviews and to diffuse tension before it balloons into misunderstanding.

This section acknowledges that engagement is often uncomfortable, not necessarily obvious, and rarely easy to nurture. "Understanding and Respecting Values" points out that true collaboration requires that we blend different perspectives on personal responsibility, fairness, and the role of government into a single voice with the power to transform health policy at the local and national levels. That's an ambitious goal, but the payoff can be significant. A case study from Scotland reveals that when citizens come to an agreement about local values, their shared commitment becomes a platform for addressing health disparities on a community level.

The chapters that follow consider relationships that are not naturally collaborative. "Traditional and New Data: Competing or Compatible?" contrasts traditional scientific approaches—such as the use of surveys and replicable research—with the new world of data science, where an explosion of real-time data is available from online platforms and social media.

"Promises and Pitfalls of Cross-Sector Research Collaboration" looks at opportunities to engage disparate players in the quest for knowledge while shining a spotlight on the data demands, language conflicts, and unpredictable environments that can create institutional silos across systems. Recognizing the value of partnerships is an essential first step, but until the partners actually learn to "play together," their path forward is likely to be rocky.

The section's final chapter, "Anchor Institutions: Harnessing Economic Power for a Healthy Community," explores how health systems, universities, and other institutions can work outside their walls to collaborate with neighborhood, employment, housing, safety, and educational organizations. Their commitment to create healthier communities is building a movement that taps into the very foundation of a Culture of Health while asking institutions to rethink the way they do business.

As this section makes clear, collaborative relationships are more the norm than ever before, and they are here to stay. As players with different agendas, constituencies, skill sets, values, and political perspectives come together, their capacity to interweave objectives, resources, strategies, and outcomes suggests a pathway toward a healthier future for all.

Understanding and Respecting Values

ERIKA BLACKSHER, PHD

Associate Professor and Director of Undergraduate Studies, Department of Bioethics and Humanities, University of Washington at Seattle

SIR HARRY BURNS, MD, MPH

Professor and Director of Global Health, International Public Policy Institute, University of Strathclyde

LARRY L. BYE, MA

Senior fellow, Health Care Research Department at NORC, University of Chicago

KATHERINE GRACE CARMAN, PHD

Economist and Professor, Pardee RAND Graduate School, RAND Corporation

MICHAEL A. RODRIGUEZ, MD, MPH

Professor and Vice Chair, Department of Family Medicine; Director, UCLA Blum Center on Poverty and Health in Latin America; Co-Director of the Center of Expertise on Migration and Health, University of California at Los Angeles

Why open a section on the power of collaboration with a chapter about values? In many ways, the answer is simple. Developing awareness of personal values and coming to appreciate the values of others are essential precursors to meaningful collaboration. We know that it will be nearly impossible to attain a Culture of Health if the nation does not acknowledge and appreciate the diverse values that contribute to a rich society. From the Robert Wood Johnson Foundation's (RWJF) own work in developing the Culture of Health Action Framework for achieving this goal, we know that valuing the best health possible for everyone and "making health a shared value" are critical components in this process.

But the topic is not an easy one to take on. The process of engaging with others and respecting their values forces individuals to deal frequently and honestly with people who see the world very differently than they do and to live different lives within it. It requires that we embrace the concept of "value pluralism" in order to work toward a greater good, and that is not easy to do.

In this chapter, contributors Erika Blacksher, Larry L. Bye, and Katherine Grace Carman paint a comprehensive picture of how uniquely American values—ranging from personal responsibility, fairness, and the scope of government authority—impact views of health policy. Contributors Sir Harry Burns and Michael A. Rodriguez enlarge that picture with an international perspective as they highlight the importance of respecting local values in a Scottish community plagued by health disparities but determined to change.

What Drives Values About Health?

Building a Culture of Health means getting to a shared value that improving health and well-being is a priority.
—*Katherine Grace Carman*

Action Area 1 of the Culture of Health Action Framework—"making health a shared value"—identifies three values that drive health: mindset and expectations, sense of community, and civic engagement. Carman summarized those values and offered some examples to illustrate how each is considered and measured:

- **Value: Mindset and Expectations**
  Example: Data from the 2015 RWJF Survey on National Health Attitudes indicate that 31 percent of people did not support policies to promote well-being. That number falls to around 16.5 percent among Hispanics and 19.4 percent among blacks, but is higher (36.8 percent) for whites.
- **Value: Sense of Community**
  Example: Findings from the RWJF National Survey on Health Attitudes indicate that adults aged 18–24 reported the weakest sense of membership in and emotional connection to community. People age 65 or older reported the strongest sense of membership and connection.
- **Value: Civic Engagement**
  Example: Data from the U.S. Atlas on General Election Turnout indicate that 28 states had a voter turnout of 50–60 percent.[1] Only Minnesota had a turnout of more than 70 percent. Data from the Current Population Survey[2] indicate that in every state except Utah, less than 40 percent of respondents said they engaged in volunteer activities. In Utah, between 40 and 50 percent did so.[3]

The American Health Values Survey

To understand how Americans value health and the role values play in promoting a Culture of Health, Bye presented selected findings from the 2016 American Health Values Survey, a national survey of more than 10,000 Americans.

Bye used two continua to report how respondents felt: the importance of health in their everyday lives and their beliefs about the role of government in the health arena. Detailed analyses of the survey appear in the American Health Values Survey final report[4] and in a chapter in the first volume of the Culture of Health book series, *Knowledge to Action: Accelerating Progress in Health, Well-Being, and Equity.*[5] Brief highlights of Bye's typology are presented here.

Along the two continua, survey respondents fell into one of six groups:

- **Health egalitarians** (23 percent) are less concerned than others about health in their everyday lives and favor a strong role for government in health.
  - They are likely to be concerned about health equity, but less likely to believe that disparities exist or that social determinants play a strong role in health.
  - They tend to be female, younger, of lower socioeconomic status, and white.
  - They are the least likely to vote and are politically moderate.
- **Committed activists** (18 percent) find health to be important in their everyday lives and are strongly committed to an active role for government.
  - They believe that disparities exist and that social determinants play a role in influencing health.
  - Members of this group are civically engaged and liberal.
  - They are more likely to be female, nonwhite, of lower socioeconomic status, and live in areas of high minority concentration.
  - Committed activists "have everything lined up in terms of a Culture of Health vision and in terms of concern about population health and health equity," Bye said.
- **Disinterested skeptics** (17 percent) are the least personally health conscious and do not favor a strong role for government.
  - They are skeptical about population health and health equity and are not likely to be civically engaged.
  - Members of this group tend to be young, male, and conservative.
  - Among the groups that do not favor a strong role for government, there is the opportunity to engage with people in this group around private sector action in community health building, Bye said.

- **Equity advocates** (16 percent) are less concerned about health in their everyday lives, and they favor a strong role for government. "There is a very distinctive sociopolitical profile to this segment," Bye said.
  - Members of this group are civically engaged but feel less efficacy in terms of bringing about change.
  - They believe that disparities exist but are less likely to believe that social determinants affect health.
  - They are more likely to be black, educated, upscale liberals, and live in cities and suburbs.
- **Private sector champions** (14 percent) have high concern about health in their lives. They are uncertain about the role of government, but favor a strong role for the private sector.
  - This group is conflicted about the Culture of Health agenda and the role of government in health.
  - They are the least trusting of science and of the health care system.
  - They are the oldest of the six groups, and tend to be female, conservative, and of lower socioeconomic status.
- **Self-reliant individualists** (12 percent) have high concern about health in their lives and favor only a limited role for government, preferring that the private sector assume responsibility.
  - They are less likely than the other groups to be concerned with equity, solidarity, disparities, and social determinants.
  - They are the most likely to believe that people can make decisions without the need for experts.
  - This group is likely to be white, male, slightly older, and of higher socioeconomic status.

Values and Social Determinants of Health

I have started to talk about social values as the fundamental causes of health disparities.

—Erika Blacksher

Social values function as a social determinant of health, according to Blacksher. A 2008 report from the World Health Organization's Commission on the Social Determinants of Health[6] identifies social and cultural norms as one of three factors driving social determinants (the other two are governance and policy).

The Institute of Medicine's National Academy of Medicine 2013 report *Shorter Lives, Poorer Health* asks, "Is there a common denominator that helps explain why the United States is losing ground in multiple domains at once?"[7] The authors identify five contributing American social values: individual freedom, free enterprise, self-reliance, the role of religion, and federalism. "The potential relevance of these societal values cannot be ignored in attempting to explain the U.S. health disadvantage," the report concludes.

Blacksher commented on two values that are particularly important in population health policy—views of individual responsibility and beliefs about fairness—and described the use of public deliberation as a tool to explore these and other values.

Individual Responsibility

Attributions of individual responsibility for health outcomes can eclipse the role of social conditions and their contribution to outcomes. "In eclipsing, they can exculpate social conditions, social structures, social responsibility, and society at large," said Blacksher.

There are different ways to interpret "responsibility," but the tendency in America is to default to a liability or blame model. Studies have found that people are somewhat reluctant to attribute blame for poor health on the basis of race, but they are quick to place blame on the basis of behaviors. While personal liability does have a role in health outcomes, so, too, does collective responsibility, Blacksher asserted.

Fairness

The beliefs Americans hold about what is fair significantly influence their views on strategies to promote health, including the allocation of resources among groups of people, according to Blacksher.

One study found that 70 percent of Americans believe strongly that there should be equality of opportunity, but only 30 percent believe there should be equality of outcome. "I think part of the challenge is conveying to the American public the degree to which social conditions contribute to health outcomes," said Blacksher. Health behaviors matter, but it is also important to discuss the ways in which social conditions contribute to health behaviors, she emphasized.

> *Considerations of fairness shape American policy preferences to a surprisingly strong degree, and Americans have very different interpretations of what is fair.*
> —*Erika Blacksher*

Public Deliberation: A Strategy for Exploring Values

Public deliberation (or participatory deliberation) is a process in which "people come together with nonpartisan, unbiased information about a set of policy questions that pose some important social challenges," according to Blacksher. The idea is for them to take the time to talk, reflect, and learn together, and then unite around recommendations.

A carefully constructed process of public deliberation, Blacksher said, enables the creation of "deliberative spaces for people to talk with fellow Americans about what their values are and to create spaces for learning, co-learning, and transformation in values." Convening people in deliberative and intentional conversations gives them the opportunity to learn together by framing an issue as a collective challenge, creating opportunity to learn about the issues and one another's values, and developing policy preferences that are informed, considered, and public-spirited.

Already widely used in the United Kingdom, public deliberation is beginning to gain traction in the United States as well. In a controlled trial of deliberative methods, researchers found that they increased people's knowledge about a complex topic and that people from different racial, ethnic, and educational backgrounds learned and valued the opportunity to talk with one another.

> *It is important not just to talk, but to actually give people the opportunity to learn about an issue and talk with one another about an issue.*
> —Erika Blacksher

There is also promising evidence that public deliberation sticks, according to Blacksher, and that it helps people work through value differences. If people can resolve differences by accepting that value pluralism is inevitable and often a good thing, they can agree on doing something in their community that, while it helps improve health, is motivated by different reasons.

One audience member responded to Blacksher's talk with the suggestion that public deliberation be more widely used by elected officials. Too often, meeting agendas are so packaged, with the topic changing so frequently, that there is little time to really listen and learn. "That is not the way a deliberative process works, and we might practice a bit of that process in the community health work we do," he said.

In one example, legislators in a rural state convened for a four-day retreat with the goal of producing better health policy. In subsequent meetings, they discussed values, leadership, and systems thinking, and then debated various ways to invest public funds to achieve different outcomes.

Reflections on Values

Carman opened the audience discussion by asking Blacksher and Bye to reflect together on ways to harness values for social progress.

Value Pluralism

Value pluralism is healthy and good for democratic societies, Blacksher said, but people need opportunities to explore their values with others who see things differently. Through deliberative and open processes, people can come to realize that others don't lack values; rather, they simply have different values. "I think respect can be built by understanding that we are morally serious people. We have values, they just may be different," Blacksher believes.

It is also important to understand the distribution of values across issues, added Bye. There is evidence that there is broader consensus on equity in the health area than in some other policy areas. For example, he said, "If you look at the attitudes that Americans have about social welfare and income redistribution, you see more polarization and more fixed views."

> *It is a process of self-discovery that is important, and actually engaging with others whose values might be different.*
> —Erika Blacksher

But value differences about health do emerge when people start digging into the details, according to Blacksher. When the discussion moves away from individual behavior and toward creating healthy communities or addressing social determinants, the conversation is no longer solely about health. That is when things get complicated, with a lot of value heterogeneity and gridlock.

"I think we ought to prioritize issues where we think we can find common ground from people across the political spectrum," suggested Blacksher. For example, she said, promoting the well-being of young children seems to be a widely shared value across much of American society, and work in that area might engage people who do not agree on other policy issues.

"I think we have started to see the upper limits of what we can get from intervening for the children separate from the claims of their parents," countered Charles Homer, MD, former associate professor at the Harvard T. H. Chan School of Public Health and former deputy assistant secretary at the Department of Health and Human Services. He asked whether there were ways to leverage the shared values behind helping children to create broader communities of health. Another participant agreed on the need to look not only at the "innocent infant everyone is happy about helping," but at helping their parents as well.

A concern about health equity appears to drive support for an active role for government in health, Bye said. The largest group in his American Health Values Survey—the health egalitarians—"does not have a terribly distinctive political or demographic profile compared to the other groups . . . but it has a notion of health equity."

Bye is replicating the American Health Values Survey in five states, with an eye toward learning whether there are opportunities in communities to work in a less partisan and polarized way.

Values and Self-Interest

Values are supposed to be drivers, but Bruce G. Link, PhD, MS, distinguished professor of sociology and public policy at the University of California, Riverside, asked about the extent to which self-interest can overwhelm a person's values. If people apply values flexibly within some overarching principles, aren't they likely to be driven by personal interest? Public deliberation might be effective "in the moment, but when interests get involved, people revert to their interests, and the interests aren't supposed to be the drivers," he said.

Patricia A. Jennings, PhD, MEd, associate professor at the University of Virginia Curry School of Education, raised the related issue of whether values change depending on a person's situation. She recalled seeing people who had opposed the Affordable Care Act later show up at town hall meetings to protest its repeal. "Once you have something and it is taken away, your value system is different than when you don't have the thing," Jennings said.

There is a general assumption that self-interest is the prime mover in policy preferences, said Blacksher, but studies have found that "notions of fairness and other values that are not based on self-interest actually do motivate and do underpin people's policy preferences." Self-interest plays a role, she noted, but perhaps not as much of one as people generally think it does.

A View From Abroad: Valuing Communities and Residents

The concept of engaging with others and respecting values is not limited to individuals or small groups. Indeed, entire communities have started to recognize these as essential tools for working together to meet health care goals.

To illustrate this point, Rodriguez introduced an international perspective to the Culture of Health, noting that Burns's experience in Scotland challenges the rest of us to value the ability of local communities to identify problems and create solutions. "It is only fitting that we reflect on the power of local folks to make a difference, and for the rest of us to be a part of that change," Rodriguez said.

Early in his career as a hospital physician serving "the poorest parliamentary constituency in the United Kingdom," Burns realized that his patients needed more than a surgeon. They needed a public health expert who understood the "biology of social inequality"—that is, the role that circumstances such as poverty and substandard housing play in poor health outcomes. Burns returned to school for training in public health.

In Scotland, as in the United States, people are told they are unhealthy "because we smoke too much and eat the wrong kind of food," Burns said. "And if only we would 'man up' and do the right things, we would be healthy. But that is not the case—not the case in Scotland anyway," he added.

> *Fundamentally, Scotland's poor health is a reflection of the health of the poor.*
> *—Sir Harry Burns*

The Slope Index of Inequality

Data have shown that life expectancy in Scotland has not improved as much it has in other European countries. Additional data comparing life expectancy of the wealthiest 20 percent of Scotland's population with that of the poorest 20 percent demonstrate that health inequities start early in life and are accompanied by inadequate education, loss of efficacy, diminished self-esteem, and other problems.

Conditions described in the opening plenary reminded Burns of Calton, a poverty-stricken neighborhood in Glasgow. Life expectancy for a man living in Calton is 54 years, compared with a life expectancy of 67 years for an Iraqi man, he said.

Using data from the "slope index of inequality," one of two major indices to measure socioeconomic inequalities in health, Burns looked more deeply into the conditions in Calton. Examining mortality rates for each five-year age cohort, he found that mortality increased between ages 10 to 15, reached its highest level by age 30, and began to drop after age 45. The two cohorts with highest mortality—young and middle-age people—are barely affected by heart disease. Causes of death among these people are "drugs, alcohol, suicide, violence, and accidents," Burns reported.

Going Local to Create Wellness

Echoing Raj Chetty's observations about the effects of neighborhood on a child's future (refer to Chapter 2, *How Location Influences Upward Mobiliy and Health*) and citing literature on adverse early childhood experiences, Burns argued for citizen-driven action at the local level: don't wait for the government to fix things, get people to fix things for themselves. With guidance and support, community residents are capable of understanding data and using data to generate ideas and test solutions to community problems.

Burns spearheaded an initiative to do just that, aiming to "transform child-hood in Scotland," community by community. Twice each year, Burns and colleagues brought together about 800 people representing every county in Scotland. The goal was to develop ideas that would build health by focusing on what Burns called "health assets"—factors or resources that enhance the ability of individuals and communities to maintain their health and sustain well-being.

Between meetings, participants returned to their communities, tested the ideas, and tracked progress. They reported results at the next meeting. Some 1,500 ideas were tested, 40 of which produced "significant changes," according to Burns. Within three years, Scotland realized an 18 percent reduction in still-birth rates and a 15 percent reduction in infant mortality, for example. "We don't know which of those changes is most effective, and to be honest, we don't really care," said Burns. "It is moving the whole system."

Going forward, Burns plans to study the impacts of health assets and health inequality in specific places with the goal of targeting resources and establishing systems that better respond to community needs.

> We need to move from a position where local government is a provider of services and citizens see themselves as recipients, to a place where citizens are confident that they can do things and know they will get the support when they need it.
> —Sir Harry Burns

Traditional and New Data

Competing or Compatible?

MOLLYANN BRODIE, PHD, MS

*Senior Vice President for Executive Operations and Director for Public Opinion and
Survey Research, Kaiser Family Foundation*

THOMAS GOETZ, MPH, MA

Co-Founder, Iodine; Chief of Research, GoodRx

BRIAN C. QUINN, PHD

Associate Vice President, Research-Evaluation-Learning, Robert Wood Johnson Foundation

Surveys and studies that are valid, reliable, and representative provide important empirical evidence about complex policy issues. They have a long history of gauging public opinions, informing planning, and contributing to conclusions that are carefully reviewed and published in scientific literature.

But in recent years, the explosion of real-time data from Facebook, Google, Twitter, and other social media has rearranged the playing field on which information is generated, ideas are developed, and actions are taken. Rapidly constructed online surveys may generate hundreds of thousands of responses within a day or two.

These developments challenge our thinking about how knowledge is acquired and made actionable and drive us to ask how traditional and new analytic methods can be combined to the advantage of both. What can academic researchers and social media entrepreneurs learn from one another? Is there a win-win option in which large datasets can be generated quickly, pass muster for rigor, and be analyzed by people with varying levels of technical knowledge? When it comes to new and traditional data and methods, are we more inclined to see them as competing or compatible?

With this volatile state of affairs as context, contributors to this chapter—one an academic researcher and one a social media entrepreneur—explored the strengths and limitations of both well-established methods of generating evidence and the newer, increasingly popular methods available from social media and technology.

Building Bridges

The new data science world tends to operate in parallel with the more traditional social science world, and frankly, I think the two worlds sometimes look askance at each other.

—Brian C. Quinn

Brian C. Quinn, the workshop moderator, opened the session by noting that the research questions to advance a Culture of Health will be answered through cross-sector work that blends new data and methods with those that have worked well in the past. Defining the workshop goal as finding ways to build bridges between the two worlds, Quinn challenged the audience, "We need a better understanding of the nature of the problems we are up against and the potential for various solutions to help us move forward."

Probability-Based Surveys: A Traditional and Tested Method

A high-quality survey can tell you a lot about a population.
—Mollyann Brodie

Mollyann Brodie has a history of designing, conducting, and analyzing probability-based surveys. This method, she said, "provides information about what a group of people did, thought, believed, and knew, and about how those things are related." These surveys also offer insights into the relationship between opinion and action—exploring, for example, whether people act on their opinions or change their opinions based on their actions.

Researchers using probability-based surveys devote significant effort to ensuring that survey results from a random sample allow them to confidently draw conclusions about the whole group. This attribute is "the promise of a well-constructed, traditional survey research project," said Brodie.

The Affordable Care Act (ACA) illustrates how probability-based surveys can be used. After the bill became law, said Brodie, everyone wanted to know who was enrolling in the health care options that had become available. Among the many questions explored through surveys:

- Why would someone be or not be covered?
- Do demographic characteristics account for variation in coverage?

- Did people's opinions of the act affect whether they sought coverage?
- Did people understand the penalties for not enrolling in an insurance plan?

The survey provided insights into the relationships between people's opinions and their knowledge, health status, demographic status, and experiences. "The study generated a lot of data that helped people understand the dynamics of the early years of the Affordable Care Act," she concluded.

But there can also be a downside to probability-based surveys, as Brodie experienced in her analysis of the ACA: they take a long time to conduct, response rates are sometimes low, and they rely on self-reports of behavior, which might not be accurate. For example, many survey respondents had received insurance premium subsidies under the act, yet all said they had not.

A Fit-for-Purpose Framework

Brodie envisions a future in which traditional research methods combine with newer methods based in data science and digital tracing. "Just think about what I could have learned," she says, by combining survey data with administrative data and information about the structure and cost of insurance plans. That combination would have provided insights into patterns of health care utilization and health status while data from geocoding would have revealed where people went to enroll for coverage.

While committed to a "fit-for-purpose" research framework, Brodie believes that two forces will compel continued attention to traditional analytic methods: first, most questions of public policy will be answered by datasets that combine measures, harnessing traditional survey research with big data and data tracing tools; and, second, as long as datasets do not include everyone in a population, "we are going to have to have benchmarks, to tell us how our study population looks compared to the whole group we want to talk about," she said.

Current benchmarks such as the American Community Survey of the Census Bureau, the National Health Interview Survey of the Centers for Disease Control and Prevention, and the multiple Bureau of Labor Statistics surveys, for example, will be imperative for the foreseeable future.

New Methods From an Experimenter, Not an Expert

We have a great body of research around what works in highly controlled environments. But then we release treatments into the wild and we don't have a good way of understanding how they work, what happens to them.
—Thomas Goetz

Thomas Goetz works with data generated exclusively online, with the goal of improving what happens when "we release treatments into the wild."

Goetz is cofounder and chief executive officer of Iodine, a digital health company that combines patient experience with medical research to help people make health decisions, generally about their medications. *Entrepreneur* magazine named Iodine one of the Most Innovative Companies of 2016. Goetz describes himself as "not an expert so much as an experimenter" in exploring new methods for translating knowledge to action.

Iodine aims to understand and communicate which medications patients prefer and whether they perceive a medication as "worth it." "Scientists or researchers will ask 'What does "worth it" mean?'" observed Goetz. "And we say it means whatever people want it to mean, because 'worth it' is a way we describe lots of things."

In one real-world test, clinical trials had found two medications for renal cancer to be equally effective. "Drug A" was prescribed more often because it had been approved before "Drug B." Researchers divided patients into two cohorts, each taking one of the drugs, and later switched the drugs, so that all patients had experience with both drugs. Patients much preferred Drug B because it was much easier to tolerate, contradicting typical prescribing practice. "What do we do with that kind of information?" asked Goetz. "Do we change practice, educate doctors?"

New technology and new techniques provide an opportunity to ask questions at scale, to gather subjective experience at scale, to measure and quantify it and work it into our practice. That is not replacing—it is augmenting—clinical effectiveness.
—Thomas Goetz

Goetz used new technology to jump-start his company. Iodine sought to learn about the experiences people have with medications but did not want to launch with "a blank website that simply asked people to share their experiences," he recalled. Instead, the company posted a short survey on Google Surveys, collected more than 100,000 viewer reports on medications, and was able to open its website at scale. Google Surveys are "remarkably accurate" at scale, noted Goetz, with their findings enriched by the capacity to infer respondent demographics and other attributes.

As former Entrepreneur in Residence at the Robert Wood Johnson Foundation (RWJF), Goetz worked with researchers at a school of public health on a project that involved both a traditional survey company and Google Surveys. "The researchers . . . were reluctant to use Google Surveys because it wasn't their typical course of action," Goetz recalled. A challenge, he believes, is finding ways to describe these new instruments to help traditional researchers recognize them "as appropriate and as valid as all the other things that we have great names for, like randomized controlled trials."

The Complexity of New Data and Methods

Big data has the potential to expand the amount and type of information available for analysis and can be mined by a growing cadre of talented researchers throughout the world. The potential for that kind of global connectivity could lead to new collaborations and break down silos across disciplines.

But because so many people can access, download, and analyze data, "we run a real risk of junk science and the risk that junk science will eliminate all faith in science," cautioned Goetz. Another concern is that the allure of vast new data and cutting-edge technology for commercial gain or trivial entertainment will drown out attention to their use to generate knowledge and solve important problems.

Organizations can and do use data captured from social media to inform policy, but researchers and data experts have access to that data as well and could conduct further analyses or even download the raw data to run their own experiments. Big data has multiple uses: it allows people to learn and to test hypotheses or interventions, but it also allows them to create algorithms that speed up automation. These uses overlap, but they are not the same and they need different analytic techniques, which can be employed by people with different backgrounds and interests.

Reflections on Data and Methods

Audience members further explored issues raised by the presenters.

Roles for Foundations

Quinn asked presenters about what a foundation could do to build on the promise of integrating traditional and new approaches, commenting that RWJF "does not get a lot of proposals that merge these two worlds."

Goetz applauded RWJF's interest here and urged the Foundation to educate other funders and tell researchers dealing with new data that it is open to funding their ideas. "I don't think people who have these skills think 'I should apply for a research project' when they think they know only how to write algorithms about text messages," Goetz observed. People working with these data may also be unsure what problems need to be solved and would benefit from working with researchers who have experience in using data to address important policy issues.

The hurdle goes in both directions because people immersed in traditional approaches may not have the expertise to use new data skillfully. "I don't have a clue how these guys do their work," Brodie admitted. "I can see what I might want to do, but I have no ability to get from here to there."

Goetz noted two promising systems-based projects that work with new data and methods. Through MakerNurse, an RWJF-supported initiative, a community of inventive nurses is working to create solutions that will improve patient care. In another initiative, Eric Hekler, PhD, of Arizona State University received support from both the National Science Foundation and Google to advance "agile science"—personalized and precise behavior change interventions that draw on new and emerging technologies.

Making Sure That Everyone's Voice Is Heard

> My purpose is to give voice to the public and to people who don't have a
> voice. They have to have a voice in my survey data.
> —Mollyann Brodie

A significant concern is that some groups of people are not included in the big datasets. Phone apps that record air quality, physical activity, or sleep patterns capture data only from people who have smartphones that feature those apps. The experiences of those without access to such features will not be captured, and their interests will not be considered by researchers or policymakers. This is where traditional methods of representative sampling are important.

Will Representative Sampling Endure?

One audience member argued that representative sampling in health research is on the wane. If a convenience sample of 500,000 people respond to an online survey, it is hard to argue the merits of a representative sample gathered through traditional methods that surveys only 2,000. The challenge, he described, is "ultimately we are going to have to find a way to reweight from the weird convenience samples."

One of the biggest challenges is transparency, according to Brodie. Many people are not ready to share the details of their models or acknowledge that their modeling is study-specific. This is less critical if there are also alternative good measures, such as Census data. But when such measures don't exist,

Brodie warns, "we have seen big problems, especially on attitudes about race in America. That is one of the areas where modeling doesn't work."

Data Standards and Data Science

Matthew Trowbridge, MD, associate professor and associate research director, Department of Emergency Medicine and Department of Public Health at the University of Virginia, sparked a lively conversation by recounting the story of a friend who used anonymized cell phone pings to track community behavior. "I realized, 'We were no longer in a world of representative data. We had *the* data,' but little idea what to do with it."

Perhaps, someone suggested, a group of people who work with very large datasets could help create standards for people who work with social media data. Standards provided by the American Association for Public Opinion Research to people conducting traditional surveys could be a model. Seizing on this idea, Trowbridge asked, "Is there room or appetite for funding more basic standardization research?"

One participant noted that the use of the term "data science" by private industry differs from how it is used by researchers, such as those attending the conference, and that industry's appetite for risk may be higher. If something doesn't work for a commercial enterprise, data scientists can change the underlying algorithm, but that may not be an option for researchers or policymakers trying to improve health and well-being. Corporations often view data about people using their products as a means to increase their customer base, while public health officials rely on data for entirely different reasons.

Perhaps there are different standards for each use? Corporate leaders have a set of ethical responsibilities about running algorithms that have the potential to shift things at nanosecond pace, while health researchers have a very different set of ethical responsibilities.

The fit-for-purpose framework, noted Brodie, holds that researchers have to determine what they want to measure, solve, or affect. Different data, standards, and methods are involved in trying to help patients have a bigger voice in the health care system than in trying to promote sales on Amazon. Brodie worries, though, "that the shiny, flashy things will crowd out" other priorities.

Speaking from the perspective of corporations, Goetz noted that one positive aspect of new and nontraditional science is an increase in code and data libraries. Facebook, for example, has open-sourced its library. Although the library was developed to prompt people to click on Facebook, it is open to everyone and to being used in innovative ways, including promoting health. Part of what makes it possible for social scientists to take advantage of data science is that the code libraries are in essence "Legos for science that people can build on," Goetz said.

Goetz's company has benefited from this resource. People who take multiple pills can easily forget what they have taken or take the wrong pill. For some time, Iodine had been trying to help people take pictures of their pills as a way to reduce those errors, and, when Facebook released its facial recognition codes, "that put us a year ahead," recalls Goetz.

Some companies become research and development hubs, collecting massive amounts of community and social data, but their data do not then come back out to communities. One participant suggested there might be a place for corporate–researcher partnerships that would help corporations share data to advance public health.

Another participant said that while there might be new sources of data and new uncertainties about reliability, validity, or representatives, there are not new data problems. Big data is just more data, he suggested. Goetz agreed that the basic structures are common, but "you get exponential complexity when you start to build in more noise and things like that, and I think it is often hard for traditional structures to grapple with that noisiness and messiness."

Working Together: Collaborative Relationships and a Dose of Humility

The tensions between new and traditional data are similar to tensions that have arisen in other kinds of interdisciplinary groups. One audience member asked if there were best practices from other disciplines that might help bridge the gap. "As a young researcher, I am often a translator because I came of age using both traditional methods and Twitter and Facebook."

Brodie noted that some firms, data scientists, and traditional researchers understand that there are pluses and minuses to each method, while others do not. Mutual respect and a sense of humility are essential to forging these relationships, she said.

A Final Word

In the current environment, evidence and data are too often weapons of ideological warfare rather than thoughtful resources for debating solutions to complex problems. Accusations that evidence is manufactured or manipulated by out-of-touch researchers and irresponsible journalists have raised deep concerns among the American people that information, no matter its source, can no longer be trusted. As the contributors and participants to this discussion confirm, the worlds of new data science and traditional social science can no longer afford to look askance at one another. All of them stand to benefit from collaboration that integrates traditional and new data approaches with an eye toward compatibility, not competition.

Promises and Pitfalls of Cross-Sector Research Collaboration

JESSICA ALLEN, PHD

Joint Deputy Director, Institute of Health Equity, University College London

KACIE DRAGAN, MPH

Lead Analyst, Robert F. Wagner Graduate School of Public Service, New York University

LISA DUBAY, PHD, SCM

Senior Fellow, Health Policy Center, Urban Institute; Co-Director, National Coordinating Center for Robert Wood Johnson Foundation's Policies for Action

SANDI L. PRUITT, PHD

Assistant Professor, Department of Clinical Sciences, University of Texas Southwestern Medical Center

CORIANNE SCALLY, PHD

Senior Research Associate, Metropolitan Housing and Communities Policy Center, Urban Institute

MICHAEL S. SHAFER, PHD

Director, Center for Applied Behavioral Health Policy, and Professor, College of Public Service and Community Solutions, Arizona State University

As the interwoven connections between health and other social arenas become more apparent and accepted, cross-sector collaborations among researchers, practitioners, community organizations, and policymakers are increasingly the norm. Combining data and analyses, these endeavors hold great promise but must also confront the complexity of disparate data demands, language conflicts, and the unpredictability that characterizes the environment today.

This chapter looks at how that is being done. It draws first from U.S. contributors—grantees of the Robert Wood Johnson Foundation's (RWJF) signature research programs—who provide a clear portrait of the benefits and demands of cross-sector research. Their varied examples include a community–academic partnership to study the impact of community-based food distribution on the health and financial security of food bank clients; partnerships between health care and housing providers; collaborations among academic researchers from different disciplines and public agencies to use Medicaid data to investigate the impact of non-health policies on health outcomes; and working groups of people affected by mental illness, payers, advocates, providers, and researchers to improve behavioral health care services for high-risk individuals.

That is followed by a description of the Pan American Health Organisation Commission on Equity and Health Inequalities, an international endeavor. The commission is gathering cross-sector data and policy impact studies to understand health inequalities and actions to reduce them in 15 countries in North, Central, and South America.

The chapter offers lessons and insights from each of these efforts and points to the power of relationship-building that underlies successful collaboration across research sectors and between research and other sectors, at local, national, and international levels.

Health and Food Insecurity Among Food Bank Clients

Sandi L. Pruitt is codirector of the Community Assistance Research initiative (CARE), a multisector partnership between community stakeholders and academic researchers designed to improve the lives of low-income households in Dallas County, Texas, through evidence-based research. With support from RWJF's *Evidence for Action* signature research program, CARE seeks to understand health and food insecurity among food bank clients. *Evidence for Action* supports studies that address gaps in knowledge needed to inform, develop, and refine strategies to build a Culture of Health.

Current research has produced good information on who is food insecure and the health needs of that population, according to Pruitt. But most research is based on national survey data or on data from the Women, Infants, and Children nutrition program (WIC) or the Supplemental Nutrition Assistance Program (SNAP).

Data from the food banking sector are sparse, yet these data are especially important for understanding and mitigating food insecurity since many people who are food insecure are either ineligible for SNAP or do not access it for another reason (e.g., being undocumented or distrusting the government).

CARE's community–academic partnership includes several sectors "joined under the common purpose of identifying where the data needs are to better improve the health of people who are food insecure," Pruitt explained. These are:

- Nonprofit food assistance providers:
  - North Texas Food Bank, one of the largest food banks in the United States, with a catchment area that includes 13 counties in North Texas.
  - Hunger Center of North Texas, the food bank's research arm. Many food banks do not have a research arm, so this means, said Pruitt, "that we're starting from a place of collaboration, interdisciplinary understanding, [and commitment to] the importance of research."
  - Crossroads Community Services, the food bank's largest food distributor. Crossroads was an early developer of a computerized algorithm that calculates the right amount of food to meet each family's nutritional needs, as determined by the number, age, and gender of family members and whether someone is doing labor, such as construction, and requires a higher caloric intake.
  - Crossroads distributes food through its in-house pantry and about 60 community distribution partners across Dallas County (including public housing facilities, churches, and community centers). Dallas County covers 880 square miles, with almost 500,000 residents considered food insecure (one in five, and one in four children).
- An interdisciplinary team of professors and students from University of Texas at Dallas, University of North Texas, and University of Dallas that includes an economist, medical anthropologists, a psychologist, and a mathematician.
- Health researchers and a physician from the University of Texas Southwestern Medical Center.

The research team is tracking a range of outcomes over time among individuals visiting Crossroads distribution sites. One of the most important measures is body mass index. "Contrary to what many people think, there are not a lot of food-insecure people who are underweight," stressed Pruitt. "Less than 1 percent of our sample is underweight, 41 percent is obese, and a startling 15 percent is morbidly obese." The team has already published two qualitative and formative manuscripts documenting the primary health needs of Crossroads clients.[1] Their *Evidence for Action*–funded work will leverage longitudinal, multisector data to understand how community-based food distribution impacts clients' health and economic stability.

Building the Community–Academic Partnership

The food assistance sector and researchers have unique needs, something to offer each other, and a shared purpose:

- The North Texas Food Bank needs data for grant applications and to evaluate programming. Its research arm has de-identified data available to anyone interested in understanding more about the food banking sector and the health of people who are food insecure.
- Crossroads has regular access to, and trusting relationships with, low-income, food-insecure individuals who typically may not talk with researchers. "Crossroads also had something to gain. They wanted to know how to serve their clients better," said Pruitt.
- The researchers were excited about the quality of the data, which Pruitt describes as "clean, large, robust, and longitudinal." In return, they could offer health expertise to other team members who wanted to understand health needs but have limited knowledge about how to assess the health of food-insecure clients.

Lessons and Insights from Cross-Sector Collaboration

Pruitt cited several lessons and insights that have emerged from challenges inherent in this undertaking:

- *Language:* It is hard for one sector to learn to communicate with another sector, yet a shared language is necessary to productive collaboration.
- *Constant change:* Changes in the food banking sector (e.g., new U.S. Department of Agriculture policies and new interpretations of existing policies) altered the research design almost weekly. Researchers must be flexible and able to modify research plans and protocols to accommodate these fluctuations.
- *Time:* It is a challenge to get people to attend stakeholder meetings when they are focused on distributing large quantities of food. Sensitivity to competing time demands is required for continued progress.
- *Differences in research literacy:* "Understanding and interpreting the data is not always intuitive" for staff within the food assistance sector. "I feel like half of my time is spent educating people about what data are, what they mean, and how to use them appropriately so that findings are interpreted correctly and not misguiding any policy," Pruitt acknowledged. Likewise, understanding data collected opportunistically through food pantries, such as repeated

measurements of SNAP allotments and types of food received by clients, requires new knowledge for health researchers.

Connecting Health Care and Housing Providers

Another example of cross-sector research emerges from the Urban Institute, which serves as the national coordinating center to RWJF's *Policies for Action* signature research program. *Policies for Action* is designed to build evidence for how policies, laws, and other regulatory tools can advance the Culture of Health. Five research hubs provide transdisciplinary settings that bring together the perspectives from traditional health fields and from nontraditional areas including education, economics, transportation, justice, and housing.

Housing expert Corianne Scally described the Urban Institute's study on emerging partnerships between health care and housing providers.[2] It is being conducted by an interdisciplinary team that draws from staff across four centers—Health Policy Center; Labor, Human Services, and Population Center; Income and Benefits Policy Center; and Metropolitan Housing and Communities Policy Center. "This is a great opportunity within the Urban Institute to collaborate across our own silos," said Scally.

These partnerships are led by a health care organization seeking to align health and housing services in one location, optimize health care sector investments in housing, or promote health improvement through housing and community development policies.

The focus is on partnerships with at least one health care and one housing organization, especially those targeting families and children. "There is a very significant evidence base on the benefits of supportive housing that brings together housing plus services for special needs populations," said Scally.

Researchers interviewed some 30 experts: representatives of hospitals and health systems, payers, physicians, housing technical assistance providers, local government officials, and funders and financial intermediaries. They asked about innovative practices and how they started, who their partners were, what goals they had set, and what impact they had. Researchers also inquired about the evidence needed to evaluate success, especially around sustainability, scalability, and replicability.

The team selected six diverse partnerships for case study. Among them:

- A single hospital partnering with the city housing department and United Way.[3]

- A federally qualified health center and a nonprofit community developer engaged in both housing and workforce development in partnership with a U.S. Treasury–certified community lender.[4]
- A public health department, hospital, and public housing authority along with local and national foundations.[5]
- A national payer working with a range of housing intermediaries, local nonprofit housing developers, and service organizations throughout the country.[6]

The interventions launched through these partnerships range from integrated pest management, housing vouchers, and housing renovation, to co-location of facilities and connecting Medicaid-eligible homeless individuals with a managed care organization.

Lessons and Insights From Cross-Sector Collaboration

Scally noted some lessons and insights from these cross-sector collaborations:

- *Silos:* Real and perceived silos between the health and housing sectors proved challenging for both sides. Health-based participants viewed the housing sector as "impossible, over-regulated, and fragmented," while the housing side "accused the health care sector of being too complicated, with hospitals staying within their own four walls." Efforts to bridge the distance between them and work out solutions to difficult issues can lead to more productive working relationships.
- *Language:* The two sectors "speak different languages. Health care speaks about people, but housing speaks about units." The acronyms in both sectors are "dizzying and change often." Teaching individuals from each side the language of the other so that they can act as "translators" has been an effective way to mitigate this barrier.
- *Data integration:* Merging health data with housing data can be complicated. "Those industries have very different standards for data privacy," said Scally, adding that "it can be helpful to try to bring these together."
- *Community engagement:* Interventions were "fairly top-down," with little discussion of needs with the community. This issue is not dealt with as much as it should be, according to Scally, and can be "problematic" for a successful collaboration.
- *Leverage/funding:* The cases included very complex sets of partners. "We learned about successful ways that they were braiding financing from health care and housing sectors." Direct investments can be a "huge opportunity," since "hospitals have foundations and endowments, and payers have required reserves that vary by state as well as profits they can leverage for housing investments."

Studying the Impact of Non-Health Policies on Health Outcomes

A multidisciplinary group of researchers constitute the *Policies for Action* research hub at New York University's (NYU) Wagner Graduate School of Public Service. The hub focuses on developing innovative, practical approaches to improving the health of low-income, urban populations by measuring and connecting health outcomes to community conditions.

"Our mandate is to look at the impact of non-health policies on health outcomes," said epidemiologist Kacie Dragan, project manager for the hub. "We are trying to quantify how those policies—from sectors like housing, education, transportation—are affecting the health of low-income New Yorkers."

Through a partnership with NYU's Health Evaluation and Analytics Lab (HEAL), researchers have access to New York State's Medicaid claims database. HEAL has an agreement with the state "that says NYU can be the academic node for the Medicaid program in New York State, answering long-standing policy questions that no one has had time or resources to look into," Dragan explained.

The aim is to evaluate policies rather than programs, an effort that brings together partners from a number of NYU research centers (Center for Urban Progress, Furman Center for Real Estate and Urban Development, Institute for Education and Social Policy, and Rudin Center for Transportation), other interested faculty, and city government staff.

The Medicaid data are very rich; data from 6 to 7 million members and 200 to 300 million claims per year for seven years result in billions of data points. "We know everything," said Dragan, exaggerating only modestly: "when they go to the doctor, when they get a prescription, how much that costs. And also their welfare eligibility, if they're on food stamps, immigrants, or married."

One illustration of how these data can be used is a transportation study to evaluate New York City's Vision Zero policy, which aims to reduce traffic deaths in the city. Researchers matched data from the Taxi and Limousine Commission with Medicaid data to see if injuries and deaths related to traffic declined in neighborhoods where the speed limit decreased.

Another study, involving a partnership between NYU's Furman Center for Real Estate and Urban Development and the New York City Housing Authority, is looking at how the health of people living in public housing units is affected when the unit is renovated. They are interested, for example, in connections

> *This is a different way to go about cross-sector collaboration—starting with a really big dataset and asking our collaborators: "What questions do you need answered?"*
> —Kacie Dragan

between mold renovation and asthma, and between security improvements and mental health.

Building the Cross-Sector Research Team

The Medicaid dataset has been the "biggest asset," said Dragan. It is "such a hook for researchers from other sectors, even if they don't have any health care experience." When they hear about the sample size of 6 million, "they want to jump onboard."

The other "huge asset" in establishing a workable group of researchers was the opportunity to spend the first year with internal partners located in the same university building, with whom it was easy to communicate. After working out some kinks, the team developed a better of understanding of what they can and cannot do to answer research questions. Now they are connecting with external researchers to think about questions the Medicaid data can help answer. "We're hoping to reach out to city staff and researchers to answer some of the questions they have," Dragan said.

Lessons and Insights From Cross-Sector Collaboration

Dragan cited several key challenges in the process and lessons and insights that have been learned:

- *The dataset:* Handling the raw dataset has been the biggest challenge. Cleaning and managing billions of records across seven years has been time-consuming, resulting in a six-month lag for research-ready data.
- *Medicaid data features:* Many researchers from other sectors are not familiar with Medicaid terminology, such as ICD-10 codes or what dual eligibility for Medicare and Medicaid means. "It's a learning curve for all of us to figure out the unique features of claims data and what we can't answer because of the way it's set up."
- *Prioritization:* Currently the team is coordinating more than a dozen individual projects. Prioritizing and connecting people with similar projects is important to avoid duplication.
- *Sharing methods across sectors:* The team is contemplating a machine learning project with housing researchers that would "use big data methods, in a way that's empirically sound, to find clusters of health conditions and housing conditions." Most health and housing researchers have never worked with machine learning before, and this is one example of the considerable benefits of learning and sharing new methods.

Improving High-Risk Behavioral Health Services

People with mental illness or substance abuse typically have detectable symptoms for 8 to 10 years before diagnosis, according to Arizona State University behavioral health researcher Michael S. Shafer. Also of deep concern is that people with serious mental illness die 30 years prematurely, on average, partly because a mental health diagnosis tends to overshadow other diagnoses.

Arizona State University is a collaborating research center for RWJF's *Systems for Action* signature research program. *Systems for Action* seeks to discover and apply new evidence about ways to align delivery and financing systems supporting a Culture of Health. Shafer co-leads an effort "to achieve better alignment among the multisector policy players in Maricopa County [which includes Phoenix] to improve care and efficiency for high-risk behavioral health populations."

The research team's approach combines "big data action research with an active, broad stakeholder engagement strategy and high-end, advanced data integration, data modeling, and decision analysis, to accelerate consensus on policymaking," Shafer explained.

The project has four aims:

- Create an "integration quotient" for individuals enrolled in the regional behavioral health authority network. The integration quotient articulates, by individual, total Medicaid spending and behavioral health spending as a proportion of total health spending, along with the composition of services and procedures.
- Develop predictive models of psychiatric and general hospitalization focused on high cost/high-use individuals and based on pre- and post-hospitalization behavioral and physical health care utilization patterns.
- Develop predictive models of criminal justice system involvement focused on frequent users of care and based on behavioral and physical health utilization patterns before, during, and after they connect with the criminal justice system.
- Develop visualizations of these analyses that can facilitate multisector policymaker dialogue and decision-making to establish a Culture of Health for people with behavioral health issues enrolled in Medicaid.

A group of more than 60 stakeholders meets with researchers quarterly. Members include people with mental illness, parents of people with mental illness, payers, and representatives of the advocacy and treatment communities and the criminal justice system. Three work groups address:

- *Activation and engagement*—creating a Culture of Health for this population
- *Data visualization and analytics*—gathering and interpreting data
- *Policy*—county, state, and federal policies impeding better individual outcomes

The university's Center for Health Information Research receives all Arizona Medicaid claims data. The researchers layer these data with hospital discharge data and are in the process of obtaining criminal justice system data (such as jail bookings, court disposition, and probation). Hospitalizations and jail bookings are conceptualized as "sentinel events" that reflect "adverse effects that run counter to a Culture of Health," Shafer said.

Researchers will employ the university's Decision Theater Network, a technologically supported location ("the drum") that enables the visualization of solutions to complex problems by using the researchers' data to test hypotheses in real time. "Our intent is to bring policymakers into the drum to hypothesize and visualize different policy alternatives to reduce unwarranted hospitalization and jail booking."

Bringing Systems Together

A strain between systems of care is evident in many corners, observed Shafer, "between the state policy makers and the privatized payers, between the privatized payers and nonprofit service delivery providers, and between these partners and the criminal justice system." While they may work together, he said, "they often don't play together well."

At the same time, the willingness of the criminal justice system to participate in the project has been reassuring. "They recognize that often the police/jail/court system is the system of first response and last resort in dealing with an increasingly privatized and profit-based safety net health care delivery system," said Shafer.

Lessons and Insights From Cross-Sector Collaboration

Rarely do these systems step outside their silos. If we, as a public university, can serve as the gathering force, we've made tremendous headway.
—Michael S. Shafer

The work is contingent upon the interpersonal relationships among and between the system partners and collaborators, and on the trust that has developed, Shafer emphasized. "We've been in the community for many years. It takes time to create that."

Here, too, language is a barrier. For example, the criminal justice system calls the people they work with "offenders," while behavioral health calls them "members," underscoring the need to establish a common lexicon. Given the considerable overlap between individuals experiencing significant behavioral health issues and those involved in the criminal justice system, multisector data analytics can be helpful to identify commonalities and opportunities for improvement.

But, said Shafer, it is important to limit the pull of numbers. "Our hope is to move the data from a numbers format into visualizations that can allow real-time hypothesis testing." The health care and criminal justice systems have the similar aims of limiting utilization and costs and stand to benefit from working together. "There is good evidence of the impact of specific community health and policing interventions upon hospitalization and criminal justice system involvement," he added.

For example, Shafer asks, "What if we doubled the number of assertive community treatment teams or increased the number of police officers trained in crisis intervention teams? Can we model the potential impact of these community interventions on system-specific utilization patterns?"

Shafer's hope is that collaboration "will lead to more informed and more shared policymaking on both sides of the spectrum."

An Overarching Lesson: Build Relationships to Further Collaboration

In the examples presented by the U.S. contributors, the availability of strong data is a key driver, but, ultimately, it is relationships that undergird successful collaborations. As one audience member observed, "The time necessary to build the relationships may be more important than the power of the data." Strong relationships can break down silos between sectors, help mitigate language challenges, lead to more productive sharing of data and methods, and further community engagement—all common issues for collaborative research.

With this in mind, audience questions focused on how to maximize data use and design studies that meet the needs of partners that are at times quite disparate.

Investing Time

Audience question: How can researchers not undersell the investment in terms of time, resources, and relationship-building needed to get the desired outcome?

At NYU, said Dragan, the team quantifies the amount and types of time and other inputs that go into the research projects. This includes tracking hours worked by students and interns, as well as researcher hours, and data training time. They do that "to demonstrate that, while we don't have answers [yet] to our hypotheses, we do have a lot of descriptive data and we have spent a ton of hours to get that."

The Urban Institute has historically been a much siloed organization, according to Lisa Dubay. Several years ago, the vice president for research established a number of cross-center initiatives—social determinants of health was one—to bring people out of their silos. Included in this effort was funding to support time to build relationships across the institute's centers.

"Had we not been doing that before we became a hub for *Policies for Action*," said Dubay, "we would have been at an enormous disadvantage. We would have had to build those relationships from scratch."

Reaching Stakeholders

Audience question: With very large projects, how can researchers communicate best to multiple stakeholders not just about what the data say, but also what they don't say, and what stakeholders need to think about?

Over time NYU's Dragan has learned a lot about "the limitations of the Medicaid claims data and what it can and can't do" and relays those lessons to the partners. Being aware of the problems that could arise "if we try to answer the wrong question" is critical, she said. "We have to be careful about communicating to people and being realistic."

The Urban Institute emphasizes the use of multiple dissemination strategies. "There's value in telling the same story in different ways, to different audiences, to make sure that everyone's benefiting from the knowledge you've gleaned and the shortcomings you've found." Dubay also noted that different people will pick up different strengths and weaknesses in the analysis. Training people to write as a team is a worthwhile investment.

It is fundamental in participatory action research that the people in the community under study be actively engaged in question conceptualization, data gathering and interpretation, and "bringing meaning to those data," stressed Shafer. "That principle has undergirded a lot of our work over the years." For example, his stakeholder group includes people with lived experience of psychiatric illness along with the state Medicaid director.

This is not easy, he admits. "The challenge of leveling the playing field is something I'm still learning. How do you avoid tokenism when having people from the community on the board? And how do you equip them with the knowledge and abilities to speak frankly?"

Shafer also referred to the value of including qualitative methods (e.g., extreme case sampling or an ethnographic component) along with quantitative data gathering.

State/University Relationships

Audience question: How have universities developed and maintained relationships with the state around Medicaid data access?

The relationship between NYU and New York State evolved slowly, with John Billings, JD, professor of Health Policy and Public Service at the university, initially working on a case-by-case basis. Eventually, he offered NYU as an academic hub for New York Medicaid. "It was a trust relationship that he built up over 20 years," said Dragan.

At the same time, Dragan emphasized the multiple layers of security surrounding the data, including the use of a computer not connected to the Internet that is in a locked cage and chained to a desk. "It's definitely a logistical nightmare in some sense," but necessary given the sensitivity of the data.

Other states also provide Medicaid data access to researchers. This access, said Dragan, "comes from building the relationship over time and proving that you will be candid with the research—building up the trust."

Payers and hospitals have information as well, Dragan noted, which can work for smaller scale studies. They may have interest in exploring questions about readmissions and other requirements they are striving to meet.

In Arizona, similar "iron-clad agreements are built around data use, even for exploratory work," said Shafer. He agreed that cleaning and preparing data for analysis is a significant issue, as is the surrounding security infrastructure.

Audience member Susan Buchino, PhD, OTR/L, assistant professor, School of Public Health and Information Sciences, University of Louisville, described partnerships in Ohio, Massachusetts, and elsewhere through which public universities and academic medical centers collaborate with the state Medicaid agency on developing policy and designing new approaches to health services delivery. Centers for Medicare & Medicaid Services (CMS) funds are available to match university funds through Medicaid administrative claiming. The partnership expands the capacity of the Medicaid agency to complete research and brings additional funds to the university, so the program "is a benefit to both the university and the state," she said.

Political Sensitivities

Audience question: Can state political changes affect university–state relationships related to Medicaid data access?

The state Medicaid agency is a branch of the executive office, Shafer pointed out, "so any change in the governorship could conceivably destroy the relationship. It comes back to the relationship with the governor's health policy adviser, who ultimately is going to make recommendations to the state Medicaid agency." It is critical to be responsive to the agency's information needs and to not only focus on the team's research agenda. "You ignore their needs at peril."

New York State has been cooperative in sharing data with NYU, and Dragan expects that relationship to continue. However, if "we did something totally wrong or something dangerous in releasing data, they would take it away from us in a heartbeat."

> *Relationships matter. They matter on the ground, they matter among researchers, and they matter between the researchers and the state.*
> —Lisa Dubay

Investigating Health Inequalities in Multiple Countries

The Commission on Equity and Health Inequalities in the Americas is a large-scale effort to gather evidence on health equity gaps related to gender, ethnicity, legal, and socioeconomic status across North, Central, and South America.

The commission was established in 2016 by the Pan American Health Organization (PAHO) and managed by a secretariat at UCL Institute of Health Equity and PAHO. The commission is designed to better understand health inequalities in the region of the Americas, focusing on 15 partner countries. The 13-member commission will investigate the fundamental causes of health inequities; conduct research on how social factors, gender, and ethnicity impact health; and make actionable recommendations to reduce the health equity gap.

Though an official report from the project is not due until 2018, Jessica Allen offered a preliminary look at the commission's work.

> *It's a very ambitious review. There's a strong focus on gender, ethnicity, and human rights—stronger than in previous reviews that we've undertaken—and that's a really exciting development.*
> —Jessica Allen

Three Areas of Focus, Two Overarching Principles

The countries involved in the study are Argentina, Belize, Brazil, Canada, Chile, Colombia, Costa Rica, Cuba, El Salvador, Jamaica, Mexico, Peru, Suriname, Trinidad, and the United States. "We're going to learn in depth from those countries," Allen said, noting that the cross-sector outreach will extend to civil society groups, community groups, and other contacts at international, national, and local levels. "We're working closely with them to bring in evidence, data, experiences, and qualitative information. We hope to deepen understanding of what's driving health inequalities across the whole region."

The study will assess evidence and look at case studies in three key areas:

- **Social and biological factors and the life course** (e.g., education, gender, race, ethnicity, sexuality, work, aging, and intergenerational transmission of inequality)
- **Socioeconomic and political context on two levels**
  - Macroeconomic and environmental policy (e.g., early years, fiscal policy, global economies, trade, health, and environmental issues)
  - Governance (whole government approaches, human rights protections and legislation, sustainable development goals, and building capacities)
- **Pathways to health**
  - Material circumstances (e.g., income, housing, environmental quality)
  - Social cohesion, resilience, and cultural and societal norms and values
  - Health care systems (health services and priorities, public health conditions)

Two overarching principles will inform the study:

- Health inequalities are unnecessary and unjust.
- Health inequalities can be reduced.

"There's nothing natural or inevitable about the health inequalities that we see," said Allen. "There's a certain 'normalizing' of health inequalities, but we have to keep reinforcing that they are unnecessary and that they are the result of unfair political and policy arrangements. We've got plenty of evidence now about initiatives, policies, and approaches that work and how we can build on those." Social justice programs, political empowerment, and creating economic, environmental, and social conditions for people to control their lives can all mitigate health inequity.

Rapid Changes in Health Inequality

Across the wide region under study, positive things sometimes happen very quickly, although it is not always clear why. Allen offered two examples of on-the-ground experience of significant improvement in health occurring over a relatively short period of time.

- **Aboriginal youth suicide in Canada:** Allen described the impact of two cultural supports (local self-government and land claim participation) and four community supports (health services, education, cultural facilities, and police/fire services) to reduce Aboriginal youth suicide.

  Rates of suicide were dramatic among Aboriginal youth—137.5 per 100,000 youths over a five-year study period—when there were no cultural or community supports to help create local conditions that gave young people a sense of control over their lives. But where all six supports were present, no suicides occurred within the study period.

  "Giving communities control over their own circumstances is absolutely vital in trying to improve health," said Allen. "We see this as one of the most effective approaches, and evidence of suicide among young Aboriginal people in Canada is a stark reminder of that."

- **Childhood mortality in Peru:** Mortality for children under the age of five dropped dramatically in Peru across all maternal education levels, even no education, from 2000 to 2012, for reasons that are not yet known. "We need to look at what's happened there, what has worked well, and how this is appropriate for other contexts," said Allen.

If positive changes can happen very quickly, so, too, can the opposite. Allen acknowledged the alarming increase in "diseases and deaths of despair" among middle-aged white non-Hispanic men and women in the United States from 1990 to 2010. These findings were reported by Princeton University's Anne Case, PhD, and Angus Deaton, PhD, and presented by Case at the inaugural *Sharing Knowledge* conference in March 2016.

Research Collaboration Across Nations: Another Lesson in Relationship-Building

As in the preceding U.S. examples, relationships at multiple levels are critical to research collaborations across nations. Allen emphasized the importance of finding shared goals with collaborators and stressed that many initiatives to reduce health inequalities work not only on international and national levels but also "very locally. We need to reinforce that point." In England, as an example, recent political and financial developments have elevated the importance of community-based and local approaches, rather than relying on national government bodies for action, she observed.

The Institute of Health Equity's work on these issues receives cross-party support in England when it is framed around the notion that health inequalities are unnecessary and unjust, according to Allen. Still, talking about the social determinants of health is complex, she acknowledges. Among the challenges the institute faces: communicating issues and outcomes in "anything other than a policy wonk way"; proving that solutions are cost-effective while recognizing that "we're doing this for reasons of social justice, not just financial reasons"; and creating an advocacy network to build public understanding of health inequities and the main drivers. "Politicians tell us all the time that, without public demands for action, they're not really going to act," she reports.

Allen hopes that one of the outcomes of the Commission on Equity and Health Inequalities in the Americas will be to further prioritize health inequalities across the region. "We want to make sure it's at the top of the agenda across the United Nations, across national governments, within health ministries, and on a community level to challenge some of the inequalities which they are experiencing."

A Final Word

The initiatives described in this chapter clearly illustrate the power of collaborations that engage health and non-health sectors and promote partnerships that allow communities to put evidence to productive use. A Culture of Health is possible only through the synergies that can result when ideas, data, resources, intellectual enthusiasm, and on-the-ground, get-it-done energy combine to answer complex research questions and then translate those answers into action.

As the projects illustrate, partnerships can take many forms: between academia and communities to understand and alleviate food insecurity, between health care and housing providers to meet the many needs of vulnerable populations, between health and social service systems to address behavioral health issues, and between holders of large health datasets and researchers in other social service fields. As well, they can occur at local, national, and international levels.

There are potential pitfalls, too, as partners strive to overcome differences in culture, organizational priorities, language, data literacy, content knowledge, and environmental culture. This work is not easy and requires determination and commitment, but many more opportunities are out there to be explored.

Anchor Institutions

Harnessing Economic Power for a Healthy Community

LISA JENSEN, BSN, RN

Director, Hire Local Campus Connections, Community-Campus Partnership, University of Colorado Anschutz Medical Campus

DANIELLE VARDA, PHD

Associate Professor, School of Public Affairs, University of Colorado Denver; Director, Center on Network Science

DAVID ZUCKERMAN

Director for Health Care Engagement, Democracy Collaborative

In communities across the country, a new collaborative process is taking shape. Local institutions like hospitals and universities are expanding outside their traditional roles as providers of health care and education and working deliberately to better the long-term well-being of the communities in which they reside.

That's what happened in Aurora, Colorado, after the community lost its Air Force base, its army base, and its local airport, and the Denver International Airport opened. Leaders at the University of Colorado Anschutz Medical Campus soon recognized that they couldn't sit back and watch as jobs disappeared, housing values dropped, and economic decline took hold; the strength of its own workforce and its ability to grow depended on the health of the Aurora community around it.

Instead, the campus embraced the notion that the institution had to be responsible for its neighbors' health and a partner in its community's success. With a new mission that went beyond the traditional practice of providing acute care, Anschutz Medical Campus became an "anchor institution" in Aurora.

Something similar happened in Baltimore, when 14 institutions came together to form the Baltimore Integration Partnership, a network committed to building wealth in underserved parts of the city. These 14 anchor institutions, ranging from Johns Hopkins University to Bon Secours Health System, recognized that they had a responsibility to promote employment, housing, and economic inclusiveness for a community often left behind.

The contributors to this chapter talk about how these collaborations came together as they explore the new reality of anchor institutions that harness their economic power to help create healthier communities around them.

Anchor Institutions

The concept of "anchor institutions" fits outside the box of other strategies . . .
and is really democratic in the small-d sense of the word.
—David Zuckerman

What, exactly, are anchor institutions?

According to the Democracy Collaborative, a national nonprofit based in Washington, DC. and Cleveland dedicated to developing new strategies for a more democratic economy, anchor institutions are nonprofit and public enterprises, such as universities, hospitals, and some government entities, that are rooted in their local communities by mission, invested capital, or relationships to customers, employees, and vendors. The largest and most numerous of these anchors are universities and nonprofit hospitals, frequently called "eds and meds." As place-based entities that control vast economic, human, intellectual, and institutional resources, anchor institutions have the potential to bring crucial and measurable benefits to local children, families, and communities.

In the simplest terms, anchor institutions have skin in the game when it comes to the well-being of their surroundings. The Anchor Institution Initiative reports that U.S. universities and hospitals combined spend more than $1 trillion a year, have endowments in excess of $500 billion, and employ 8 percent of the labor force. An anchor institution "can't pick up and leave," said session moderator David Zuckerman. "Because of its invested capital, because of its relationships, because of its mission, it's a lot less likely to leave its community over the long term."

An Institutional Anchor's Mission

According to the Democracy Collaborative, the mission of an anchor institution is defined as follows:

> A commitment to **intentionally** apply an institution's long-term, **place-based economic power** and human capital in partnership with community to mutually benefit the long-term well-being of both.

For a hospital or university to become an anchor institution, Zuckerman argued that it must take stock of three sets of institutional assets: functional assets (business and financing expertise, partnering capacity, training, reputation and community leadership, diversity and inclusion), economic assets (hiring capacity, supply chain and purchasing capacity, investment capacity, real estate and development), and discretionary assets (community benefit grants, community health initiatives, social and economic support services). And, he said, an institution must embrace moving beyond *individual* ownership to *community* ownership to fulfill an anchor institution's mission.

Said Zuckerman: "How do we begin to actually root our assets in place to benefit those communities? And, at the same time, how do we take an asset-based approach—and not a needs-based approach—and think about what we can leverage in that process to radically change our communities so that there's an ecosystem that is producing not only good jobs and healthy housing but ultimately health and well-being? And that is where anchor institutions come into play."

Driven by Social Determinants and the Affordable Care Act

Over the past 25 years, according to a recent survey report by the Coalition of Urban Serving Universities and the Association of Public and Land-Grant Universities, "a growing number of anchor institutions have come to realize the increasingly important roles they play in their communities and have committed themselves to greater engagement in their communities."[1] According to Zuckerman, two driving forces for health systems behind this realization stand out: greater understanding of the role social determinants play in health, and the impact of the Affordable Care Act (ACA).

Central to building a Culture of Health and as explored throughout this book, the ability to lead a healthy life begins in our homes, schools, and neighborhoods, long before we need medical care. That's evident in data about life expectancy and health disparities and how they interface with poverty, race, and place.

Zuckerman quickly highlighted some of those data. He noted that, since the 1970s, the differences in average life span after age 50 between the richest and poorest people have more than doubled to 14 years.[2] "When you parse that by race, the disparities are really dramatic," he added, showing that the net worth of whites is 13 times greater that of blacks and 10 times greater than Latino net wealth.[3] The influence of place, he said, is evidenced by the fact that the average life expectancy in a poor urban area in Ohio is 64 years, compared to an average life expectancy of 88 years in a wealthier suburban area only eight miles away.[4]

The ACA's Community Health Needs Assessment

As institutions began to recognize the impact of social determinants on health and to question their own role in building healthier communities, another critical factor emerged. An often-overlooked provision of the ACA requires every nonprofit hospital to complete a Community Health Needs Assessment in their community every three years. In a nutshell, the assessment asks: What is going on in the neighborhoods around these institutions? Do they have adequate housing, job opportunities, health care, schools, and sidewalks? As Zuckerman has emphasized in previous reports, the implementation of this ACA provision encouraged hospitals and universities to redefine themselves and their mission.[5]

The change has been intense, said Zuckerman, because institutions haven't always recognized or cared about the communities outside their institutional walls, and outreach hasn't necessarily "been in their DNA. This is about building a culture within those institutions to recognize their vested interest in seeing their community benefit because it ultimately benefits them and it's also amiably aligned with their mission."

> *It's ultimately about rethinking how we do business.*
> *—David Zuckerman*

Anchor institutions exist in every community, and there is an opportunity to get these institutions to act differently. According to Harmon Zuckerman and Ira Harkavy in *Eds and Meds: Cities' Hidden Assets*, a college, university, or medical institution is in the list of top 10 private employers in every one of the 20 largest cities in the United States.[6]

The specific directions these anchor institutions take to pursue their mission can be as diverse as the institutions themselves. David Zuckerman offered these examples in his *Hospitals Building Healthier Communities* report:[7]

- The Mayo Clinic in Rochester, Minnesota, procures from local and diverse suppliers in the area to stimulate the local economy and serves as the principal funder for First Homes, a community land trust that develops permanently affordable housing.
- Gundersen Health System in La Crosse, Wisconsin, established an aggressive program to achieve leadership in the areas of energy conservation and renewable energy, waste management, recycling, and sustainable design.
- In Cleveland, University Hospitals and Cleveland Clinic have collaborated with the Cleveland Foundation and Case Western Reserve University "to transform the city's Greater University Circle. This joint initiative expands transportation, education, and employment for the surrounding low-income neighborhoods."

According to the survey by the Coalition of Urban Serving Universities and the Association of Public and Land-Grant Universities, "Once a university embraces the anchor role, the commitment integrates itself more deeply into the urban university modus operandi. As it grows, the anchor mission may well achieve a greater integration across the university itself."[8]

Two organizations working to embrace different aspects of anchor institution missions are the University of Colorado Anschutz Medical Campus and the Baltimore Integration Partnership. Here are their stories.

A Community–Medical Campus Partnership

In 2008, the University of Colorado Health Sciences Center completed its 10-year effort to build and move its entire facility to the University of Colorado Anschutz Medical Campus, directly east of Denver in Aurora, the third-largest city in Colorado. With six health professional schools, multiple research centers and institutes, two nationally ranked teaching hospitals (University of Colorado Hospital and Children's Hospital Colorado), and the largest academic health center in the Rocky Mountain region, the Anschutz Medical Campus predicted a $3.6 billion direct economic impact on the surrounding area, reportedly greater than the Colorado ski industry.

The relocation effort had started in the late 1990s after the area's Lowry Air Force Base, the Stapleton Airport, and the Fitzsimons Army Base closed in quick succession from 1994 to 1999. The health sciences center acquired the army base located in North Aurora and proceeded to develop its one-square-mile campus in a neighborhood that was reeling from the departure of the three institutions and the resulting drop in services, property values, rental prices, and employment opportunities and a greater influx of refugees and immigrants. North Aurora's 125,000 people, with a diversity index of 86 percent and 130 languages spoken in the schools, soon reported the highest unemployment, lowest income, and lowest educational attainment ratings in the state, said session presenter Lisa Jensen.

In truth, the medical center leadership barely noticed. "As you can imagine, our institutions were very inwardly focused on funding all of this new building, providing staffing, and building the infrastructure," said Jensen. "We didn't look across the street at all except to ask that the trailer park be removed, or to have restaurants torn down. This is typical of what a lot of universities and hospitals do when they are claiming space—they move out the people living right next door."

This began to change in 2011, Jensen said, when a new chancellor named Jerry Wartgow brought his background in education and workforce development to

> *Our campus will flourish only if we become a good neighbor in the services of our neighbor's health.*
> —Jerry Wartgow, Chancellor, University of Colorado Anschutz Medical Campus

the new medical campus and its surrounding neighborhood. His assessment was decisive: a community–campus partnership was paramount.

In 2012, Wartgow commissioned a team to create a framework for a community–campus partnership with the local neighborhoods around the Anschutz Medical Campus. That, said Jensen, "is what started our journey into developing an 'anchor' mission."

A Two-Way Street: A Community–Campus Partnership

Efforts to develop a community–campus partnership on the medical campus started with the most basic steps: talking and listening to the concerns of both sides.

- In 2012, a Wartgow team member conducted some 100 "key informant" interviews with people working on campus as well as with organizational leaders in the community to understand their perceptions.
- In 2012 and 2013, an initial advisory group with representatives from both the campus and the community developed a planning committee, reviewed those interviews, and concluded they should move forward to create a community–campus partnership. The planning committee began to debate and develop vision statements, principles, goals, and programs. The signature program, everyone agreed, should be workforce development that helped local residents get jobs on the new campus.
- In the summer and fall of 2013, with funding from the Denver Foundation and the university, the planning committee officially became the Community Campus Partnership (CCP). The CCP consisted of 35 community and campus organizations, including representatives from every health sciences school and both hospitals.
- In the fall of 2014, CCP members took a field trip to Cleveland to study Cleveland's University Circle Initiative, an existing anchor institution initiative. This trip was especially important for two reasons, said Jensen. First, city officials on the trip understood for the first time the essence of the anchor institution concept. "Suddenly the lights went on in their eyes and they began to see, 'This is what we need to do,'" she said. Second, "We heard from Cleveland that one of the mistakes they made was involving the community too late. So we decided not to make that mistake."

A Community Talks, Partnership Team Members Listen

Back in Aurora during the winter of 2014, the CCP hired a community liaison to create a team of 20–25 resident leaders. This Resident Leader Council conducted what it called a "Connections Campaign"—a series of 236 interviews with local residents to listen to their concerns and identity priorities and hopes for the future. Their primary interests? Jobs and education.

At three community focus groups, participants described the barriers they faced when trying to get jobs at campus institutions. Among them, local neighborhoods were never "front and center" for campus employers looking to hire; the application process was complex and the titles and descriptions of jobs were unclear and complicated; and, more often than not, local residents lacked the required work skills, qualifications, and English-language proficiency skills.

The undisputed message from individual residents mirrored the message from community organizations: their top priority was workforce development and local jobs. The Resident Leader Council continued through monthly networking breakfasts and dinners to develop leadership skills in residents and listen to their concerns. "This helped us gain traction in the community and help people to trust that we weren't just trying to force some solution on them," said Jensen.

A Campus Talks, Partnership Team Members Listen

On the other side of the community–campus partnership, team members listened to the concerns of the campus, too. To help campus representatives understand the importance of an anchor institution, the CCP also worked to educate the campus about the community. "Campus in the Community Days" and "Community on the Campus Days" encouraged faculty and staff to venture into the community to do service learning and participate in volunteer opportunities, while community members ventured onto campus to learn about campus activities and job opportunities. An interactive website called Com-Cam.org (community-campus) provided weekly updates and newsletters about events and job opportunities that impacted both.

"This might seem small," said Jensen, "but this communication is actually helping people feel like they are a part of the campus and the campus is more aware of what's going on in the community."

Following another series of "key informant" interviews—this time with university human resource leaders and their staff—the coalition convened its inaugural Employers' Summit in June 2015. When medical campus employers acknowledged that it was difficult to hire people with diverse backgrounds from the local community—but didn't necessarily have trouble recruiting from middle- and upper-class white populations in other parts of the country—Jensen reassured them: "We can do something about this."

She explained the benefits of hiring locally and the concept of an anchor institution using its economic resources to create healthier communities. The Employers' Summit resulted in an agreement among the four main campus employer groups to meet regularly to develop and sustain a coordinated "Hire Local" effort. The drive to become an anchor institution was officially launched.

The Hire Local Program

The goals of the "Hire Local" program became establishing an accessible, reliable, and trusted Job Hub; developing an equitable, intentional, and in-clusive recruitment strategy; hiring more people from the surrounding neigh-borhoods; and supporting residents who did get hired to help them stay in their jobs, advance, and thrive in their careers. Both sides needed help to meet these goals.

With an adult basic education grant from the Colorado Department of Education, the Hire Local program in 2015 partnered with UCHealth, Children's Hospital Colorado (both are hospitals on the Anschutz Medical Campus), and Arapahoe/Douglas Works! Workforce Center to create the Healthcare Bridge Pilot Program through the Community College of Aurora. This 10-week course prepares local students for entry-level jobs in patient services on the medical campus.

By February 2017, more than 70 students had completed the program and 48 had found jobs, with a 98 percent retention rate over the first 18 months. "Obviously, we want more hires," Jensen said, "but there are aspects of this that we're very proud of."

Consider these Hire Local accomplishments from 2015 and 2016:

- UCHealth has created a "Hire Local" tab on its website, accessible when local residents apply for a job. The HR departments have not agreed to set aside jobs for local residents, but they promised to "interview everyone who comes through the Hire Local pathways," said Jensen. "That's fair. We want our can-didates to be competitive. We don't want them to be given jobs; they need to earn them."
- A special initiative works to develop job pathways for refugees and immi-grants in the neighborhoods around the medical center. Jensen noted that UCHealth tracks the number of employees they have in zip codes of interest, and she is working with Children's Hospital and the University of Colorado to add this tracking system as well.
- UCHealth hired 170 local residents, including Healthcare Bridge graduates.

- The Job Hub opened in the community in April 2017 to increase exposure to available job openings on the medical campus and is now flooded with applicants. The Job Hub also offers some intake and skills assessment to align residents with classes and resources.

Though providing jobs to local residents is at the heart of the anchor mission at Anschutz Medical Campus, Jensen concluded that establishing an anchor institution is about more than creating employment. She believes anchor institutions also build inclusivity and diversity, improve economic well-being for residents and neighborhoods alike, and enrich their own teaching, learning, clinical experiences, and research. She quoted Lilly Marks, the vice president for health affairs at the Anschutz Medical Campus, who once said, "The way to improve community health is through building community wealth." And that, said Jensen, "is what we are committed to."

Evaluating the Baltimore Integration Partnership

The value of anchor institutions and the challenges they confront are also evident from an evaluative lens. Researchers from the Center on Network Science at the University of Colorado Denver received funding from the Annie E. Casey Foundation to study the anchor initiative in Baltimore, known as the Baltimore Integration Partnership (BIP) in 2014 and 2015. Associate professor and network science researcher Danielle Varda evaluated BIP and presented her findings at the session.

BIP is one of the only multi-institutional networks (currently consisting of 14 anchor institutions) in the country. Established in 2011 as a collaborative of anchor institutions, funders, nonprofits, and public organizations, the partnership focused on establishing economic inclusion as the business culture of norm in the Baltimore region. In February 2017, the 14 anchor institutions ranged from Loyola University Maryland and Coppin State University to Bon Secours Hospital and Johns Hopkins University.

According to Varda, BIP anchor institutions have collectively agreed to focus on three goals: (1) procurement (to connect with local, small, and minority-owned businesses), (2) capital development (to leverage anchor real estate investment for the intentional benefit of the broader community and small business), and (3) workforce development (to ensure equitable opportunities and connect low-income residents to jobs within anchors).

The evaluation of this anchor initiative was based on three framing questions:

- How is "economic inclusion" implemented among anchors?

- What were the strongest and the weakest parts of the system of stakeholders that make up this effort in Baltimore?
- How is the system of stakeholders connected?

As part of the evaluation, Varda and her team sought perspectives from all parts of this complex system of stakeholders. They first interviewed 49 people at the nine anchor institutions that were then part of the partnership; followed by interviews with 61 people representing the community, including workforce development agencies, small business agencies, neighborhood associations, vendors, and residents seeking employment (primarily formerly incarcerated individuals, who represent a large proportion of the underemployed workforce in Baltimore); and completed the study with a social network survey.

Key Findings From the Anchors

In every single anchor institution, there was demonstrated commitment to this work. However, each had a different set of policies and varied on progress. The BIP was cited often as the catalyst for bringing this large group of anchors together.

—*Danielle Varda*

- **Different perspectives and definitions:** Not surprisingly, Varda found some significant variations in how BIP's anchor institutions define economic inclusion. Some defined it as simply meeting requirements, such as meeting a standard for how many contracts they give to minority- or women-owned business; other anchor institutions saw economic inclusion as a philosophy, an obligation, and a necessary component of revitalization efforts in Baltimore.
- **Achievements:** The greatest achievement of the anchor institutions, according to Varda, is a "shift in organizational culture across anchors. This is like moving a mountain. The fact that they were all committed to being around this table together and their leadership was there, talking about it, has made a big impact on progress."

  Varda also noted that BIP has connected many parts of the system. "The building of this multianchor network, working together with a common set of goals, is very dynamic," she said. "In a city that is plagued by divisiveness, especially over the course of the last few years, it is a tremendous accomplishment to have these anchors together around the same table."
- **Barriers and opportunities:** Varda identified four barriers to achieve economic inclusion that were consistent across all institutions: the ability to identify vendors, vendor capacity, an undeveloped workforce, and organizational structure limitations. One of the biggest opportunities for improvement was

integrating community perspectives on economic inclusion, which Varda suggested all institutions could do.

The Community Perspective

Capturing the community's perspective was equally important to the evaluation, but Varda and her team were warned by representatives of the anchor institutions that people might not want to participate in the project. They said, "No one will talk to you," she recalls.

"That gave us an indication that there was uncertainty from the anchor institutions about how to approach and incorporate community voice into their ongoing anchor work." In fact, quite the opposite proved true. "People were very open and eager to talk about their lives, their work, and their communities. All we had to do was call people and tell them we were interested in listening, and we were invited into businesses, homes, and community programs."

At the end of each interview, the team asked, "If you had 10 minutes in front of the anchor institutions, what would you say to them about their economic inclusion efforts?" Many responses were framed around distinct barriers resulting from structural racism and perceptions that the anchor institutions did not address some of their toughest daily challenges.

But the community's willingness to bring these issues into this conversation differed from the anchor interviews, where the focus was generally on policies and procedures being considered at their institutions, rather than on the deeper structural and systemic causes of inequity in the city. In her presentation, Varda noted one local vendor's comment that the anchors could not achieve their goals without acknowledging the causes of inequities:

A theme consistently highlighted across almost every interview is what Varda called an often overlooked "culture of helping"

> *In Baltimore city, you have to fix the issue of African-American men. Until somebody decides to do that, it's not going to matter. You got a whole generation of African-American men that have been arrested, have records, and when you drive through the city that's what you see. That's the unemployment rate of African-American men 18 to whatever, 35, 36—I mean it's ridiculous. Probably 50 percent. People want to wonder why there's so much violence and wonder why so many people are getting arrested. You're only as good as the people at the bottom. Unless somebody steps up and decides like, "We want to take this on. We're not going to be afraid. We're going to step up."*
> *—Local vendor*

and the Baltimore community's strong desire for engagement in both seeking and providing work opportunities. Across the interviews, people expressed the desire to help themselves, help each other, and help their community. They expressed gratitude that the anchors were taking on these challenges but remained skeptical that their intentions and authenticity were sincere enough to be successful.

Strengths and Challenges

When considering efforts related to procurement and capital investments, Varda heard numerous strengths (such as personal relationships, knowledge of upcoming project opportunities, mentorship, and economic inclusion in anchor institution hiring) and significant challenges (difficulty talking to anchor institutions, no system of shared resources, lengthy payment schedules, few capital resources).

The same was true of workforce development. The strengths of many anchor institutions (partnerships between agencies; serving as a conduit between employers and potential new employees to improve job placement outcomes; employer support on the job, including more educational opportunities) were offset by the same number of challenges (institutional barriers such as problematic anchor policies, socioeconomic barriers like racial stereotyping and criminal backgrounds, a lack of job awareness, or how to apply for a job with limited access to technology).

Said Varda: "Some of these policies are getting implemented without an equity lens. For example, you can increase requirements for minority-owned contracts. But what some vendors told us was that business would engage in 'fronting' or inclusion of an MBE/WBE [minority business enterprise/women business enterprise] to get a contract with work never to follow, in turn creating new racial tensions in the community. They were asking people in the community to build relationships that could *cause* more tensions than there were before that. These kinds of examples demonstrated why an equity lens that takes into account the whole system of consequences is essential to reaching anchor-specific outcomes."

Community-Driven Recommendations

In the final phase of her evaluation, Varda offered recommendations from the community that addressed both individual anchor institutions and the total BIP network. Heading the list in both categories: "include community in the decision making" and "represent communities in governance."

Varda proposed that anchor institutions reconsider who has the power to make a change and how they connect with the community. "The Baltimore anchor initiative has achieved many of its goals, starting with integrating economic inclusion policies into its practices. At the same time, any large institution is going to face barriers that make it difficult to be flexible and make quick policy changes," she added.

At a meeting in June 2017, Varda and her team invited all of the 110 participants in this work, including representatives from anchor institutions and community stakeholders, to present the findings back to them. "Our question now is, 'How do we use this information to keep the conversation going forward?'"

Reflections on Anchor Institutions

The questions from the audience revealed the challenges ahead for the growing anchor institution movement and its mission to help create healthier communities.

Funding and Upward Mobility

John Forsyth, community services administrator, Seattle Housing Authority, raised two important concerns: How do institutions get funding for these programs to prepare people to work? And is it possible for anchor institutions to help provide pathways to middle-class jobs and careers and not just entry-level positions? "We've had some success with food and environmental services jobs, but community members have said they were really interested in some higher level jobs," he said. Without upward mobility, he suggested the contribution of the anchor institution may be minimal.

Jensen noted that funding comes from multiple and varied sources— including the institutions themselves and their affiliated schools, local foundations, cities and municipalities, and workforce development organizations.

Answering Forsyth's question about entry-level jobs and upward mobility was more difficult, she acknowledged. Anschutz Medical Center employers say they need employees in food services, environmental services, and patient services, including front desk, telephone assistance, and scheduling assignments. "These pay a living wage and we were excited about focusing on that because the hospitals have a lot of need there," Jensen said. "We don't want to train for jobs that they aren't going to be hiring for."

Zuckerman observed that it is much more difficult for economic engines like anchor institutions to create a path from high school to middle-class jobs, where a college diploma is generally a criteria. However, he pointed out the progress begins by articulating the question: "How do we get these workers into frontline positions and then move them up to the middle class?"

Johns Hopkins University in Baltimore and University Hospitals in Cleveland have made a commitment by targeting recruits for entry-level positions but then creating specific pathways and timelines to move employees up. "It's very intentional," he said, pointing out that these programs have a 98 percent retention rate. "If you don't have a pathway up for those folks, your local hire strategy is only going to last so long because retention rates have spiked. And this will help your institution become more diverse."

Rural Communities: A Different Vision for Anchor Institutions

Betsy Whaley, vice president for strategic initiatives at Mountain Association for Community Economic Development, said she works with 54 Appalachian regions of Kentucky. She pointed out that these rural communities lack the anchor institutions associated with a resource-rich university system but emphasized that rural anchor institutions could be local clinics or schools or even businesses. "Is it better to start with one anchor institution or better to start with a network of them?" she asked. "What are the pros and cons?"

Jensen responded that the Anschutz Medical Center created its anchor institution from multiple medical centers, medical schools, and institutes on its campus "because it made sense to team together. It worked well, but it has its own obstacles, believe me."

Varda agreed with Whaley that local businesses can serve as anchor institutions—and pointed to a medical director of Walgreen's, sitting in the audience. "Walgreen's actually has an anchor mission and, as they say, '75 percent of the population is within five miles of a Walgreen's', making their presence in neighborhoods, as key employers and buyers of goods and services, a potential resource for community wealth building. So I think there are alternatives to eds and meds, and perhaps some of the private sector industries that have more of a presence in these places can adopt anchor-like missions of economic inclusion."

Zuckerman highlighted various online tools and reports developed by Democracy Collaborative that can help organizations analyze how well institutions work together and the infrastructure they need to carry out anchor institution missions. Two specific tools, created with funding from the Robert Wood Johnson Foundation (RWJF) and the Annie E. Casey Foundation, are:

- **Hospitals Aligned for Healthy Communities,** a toolkit series available at hospitaltoolkits.org, which includes information on place-based investing, inclusive local hiring, and inclusive local sourcing.

- **Anchor Dashboard,** which outlines key indicators that help track whether anchor institutions are making a difference and meeting the needs of the low-income communities they serve. Rural communities, Zuckerman admitted, present unique challenges and often create different definitions of wealth building. For instance, he said, the Charleston Area Medical Center in West Virginia decided to focus part of its wealth-building strategy on procuring healthy food that is produced locally, "viewing that as an opportunity to build up local farmers."

This wealth-building strategy incorporates a notion that all anchor institutions should consider, Zuckerman concluded. "It's important to keep wealth in place and not have it impacted by the whims of a marketplace. In eastern Kentucky, there was once a lot of wealth but someone picked it up and took it away. When making these investments for the next 50 years, it's important to ask, 'How do you actually make sure it stays there?'"

A Final Word

RWJF recognizes the vital role of anchor institutions as a strategy to achieve health equity. The role of cross-sector collaboration was further emphasized in a 2017 report, *Communities in Action: Pathways to Health Equity*. RWJF commissioned the report, which was the result of a year-long analysis from the National Academies of Sciences, Engineering, and Medicine, as part of a $10 million, five-year grant to examine solutions to promote health equity. The report noted that "communities have agency to promote health equity" and that "collaboration and engagement of new and diverse (multi-sector) partners is essential."

ON THE FRONT LINES
OF COMMUNITY CHANGE

Social problems and solutions look very different when they are viewed through the lens of a struggling, marginalized neighborhood rather than a classroom or conference. In settings where residents face Herculean challenges to make even incremental progress, collaboration, communication, and problem-solving are not just concepts or theory: they are the work of the day. Sometimes, academic and research principles provide indispensable guidance, but, in other situations, the practices that result can resemble the movie that doesn't translate all that well from the book on which it was based.

The three chapters in this section zero in on experiences from people on the front lines of building a Culture of Health. With case studies that feature attempts to promote equity and make meaningful change, the contributors illustrate what it means to confront the realities of vibrant but struggling neighborhoods, where residents are often too concerned with crime and living conditions, among other issues, to attend to their diabetes or ensure they eat right and exercise enough. These are stories of people who reach across disciplines and cultures and outside their comfort zones; they are also portraits of promise and rays of hope.

"Building Vibrant Communities" explores how researchers, community leaders, and residents can work together to leverage the power of local initiatives and local leaders to achieve scale and affect policies. From designing a new elementary school in a poor area of rural Virginia to reconfiguring public spaces in Kentucky and New York, contributors illustrate by example how the principles that underlie one intervention can be applied to others and ultimately have impact across a broader field. Multinational human rights treaties are put forward as a way to apply a global context to the work of both researchers and community advocates addressing social determinants.

"Bridging the Academia–Media Gap" features a conversation between a researcher and a journalist who share their perspectives about prompting community and policy change through a captivating use of the media. Held in the wake of the 2016 presidential campaign, when both evidence and journalism were being disparaged, their conversation underscores the importance of continued integrity in both professions. The contributors probe issues such as the explosion of social media; the time and resource pressures facing news outlets, journalists, and reporters; and the priorities and capacities of local newspapers.

Community activists describe their personal "Failing Forward: Pitfalls and Progress" experiences in this section's final chapter. People from organizations as diverse as a small food pantry in Maywood, Illinois, and a large hospital system in Baltimore tell honest stories about good ideas gone awry. Driven by a steadfast commitment to making a difference in their communities, all demonstrate the capacity to reflect thoughtfully on what went wrong, admit mistakes, open themselves to alternatives, and then move on to try something else.

Taken together, these chapters contribute an often missing perspective along the knowledge-to-action continuum. Here, actions on the ground inform and improve the knowledge base, revealing how insights can move in both directions. In the context of increased devolution of decision-making to states and localities, these examples are cautionary tales and helpful guides.

Building Vibrant Communities

WENDY K. MARINER

Professor of Health Law, Bioethics and Human Rights; Professor of Socio-Medical Sciences and Community Medicine Boston University School of Public Health

EDUARDO SANCHEZ, MD, MPH, FAAFP

Chief Medical Officer for Prevention and Chief of the Center for Health Metrics and Evaluation, American Heart Association

MATTHEW TROWBRIDGE, MD

Associate Professor, Emergency Medicine and Public Health; Associate Research Director, Department of Emergency Medicine, University of Virginia School of Medicine

SHIN-PEI TSAY, MSC

Executive Director, Gehl Institute

The journey toward a Culture of Health is marked by uneven steps forward, stumbles that frustrate, and, ultimately, renewed efforts backed by new knowledge and determination. It demands attention to basic human rights principles, including the right to health, endorsed by many governments throughout the world. Yet many innovative ideas never make it beyond the level of a small project or a pilot test. Few make it to scale, although scaling is an essential ingredient in connecting knowledge to action. Only through scaling do policies and interventions attain enough reach to address the structural factors that undermine health and well-being.

Eduardo Sanchez moderated a discussion among leaders representing human rights, public health, and lived experiences in public spaces. These contributors describe principles and programs that characterize the journey from testing an idea to expanding its reach. Issues of attending to basic human rights, collaborating across disciplines, and engaging stakeholders as diverse as community residents, school superintendents, and architects are explored. Short examples from the built environment and human interactions in public spaces illustrate challenges to overcome and opportunities to move forward.

Setting the Stage

Sanchez introduced the presentations by laying out the decisions that face people working on small projects with promise. "You reach that place at the end of the [test] period and questions come up," he noted. Sometimes more testing is needed because "we have not quite gotten the answer we were looking for." At other times, the intervention "works beautifully." Even here, there may not be the fiscal wherewithal or political will to take the intervention to scale, "so scaling is logistical, but it is also sometimes political and financial."

In some cases, things do not work, and program operators and researchers have to abandon a particular strategy (see Chapter 14, "Failing Forward: Pitfalls and Progress").

Strength of evidence is one element that affects these tough decisions, Sanchez observed. Others include the extent of collaboration and the extent to which cross-sector work prompts changes at the system or structural level, rather than at the program or project level.

Harnessing Human Rights on Behalf of a Culture of Health

> *Human rights explain what it means to be a person.*
>
> —*Wendy K. Mariner*

Wendy K. Mariner believes inequality and unequal opportunity violate basic human rights. As we consider how best to bring effective interventions to scale, she argues that attention to global human rights treaties creates a framework within which to harness human rights to research, policy, and practice initiatives designed to generate a Culture of Health.[1]

Multiple legal documents—the Universal Declaration of Human Rights; the International Covenant on Economic, Social, and Cultural Rights; the International Covenant on Civil and Political Rights; and others—specify rights that governments are obligated to protect. "These legal obligations by treaty just so happen to correspond to the social determinants of health," Mariner said. The overlapping concepts include standard of living; favorable and just work conditions; access to housing, food, clothing, medical, and social services; and nondiscrimination.

In "explaining what it means to be a person," human rights are indivisible and extend beyond any discipline or sector. This characteristic allows human rights proponents who may not view health as their principal goal to engage with others in building a Culture of Health. "We don't necessarily have to convince people that health is the goal in order to partner with people whose primary focus is human rights," Mariner reminded. That perspective promotes collaboration with organizations that work in education, housing, or other fields, and expands the leverage of the health sector.

A final advantage to linking human rights with a Culture of Health and social determinants of health is that human rights bring political capital to the promotion of change. Human rights principles command attention from policymakers responsible for complying with legally binding treaty obligations that have been signed by their government.

These principles are also a reminder that all people deserve respect. Despite increased attention to the social determinants of health, an emphasis on individual behavior change remains pervasive. This concerns Mariner, who observed, "It shifts our focus from improving the cards that people are dealt to telling people who got bad cards that they should play them better."

To illustrate her point, Mariner presented a list of the do's and don'ts that could theoretically influence the social determinants of health if behavior was the sole driver:

- Don't live next to a busy road or a polluting factory.
- Do own a car or live near public transport.
- Don't live in low-quality housing.
- If you are retired, unemployed, or disabled, do take all your benefits.

The advice speaks for itself: individuals do not have the ability to follow all of these admonishments; societal commitment is needed here.

Going Deep and Wide to Change the Built Environment

Two things I'm trying to figure out are how to scale by going deep in cross-sector collaborations while simultaneously thinking in terms of systems.
—Matthew Trowbridge

Matthew Trowbridge had an opportunity to move knowledge into action in Dillwyn, Virginia, as part of a team working within communities and across systems.

Home to 443 people in 2014, Dillwyn is a poor, diverse, rural community in Buckingham County. In 2009, the residents of Buckingham County had a rare opportunity to fundamentally rebuild a county primary and elementary school. "I want to do a health intervention," the school superintendent told

Trowbridge. "Obesity is a huge issue among children, and I want the school to help with that."

After realizing that his "two inches of public health articles" did not provide the right tools to build the school the superintendent envisioned, Trowbridge "went deep." His public health team engaged with the architectural design firm to do "something none of us had ever really done." Drawing from public health research, architectural principles, and the priorities of the school district, team members worked intensively to create research-based healthy eating and physical activity design guidelines for school planners, architects, and educators. The guidelines were subsequently published by the Centers for Disease Control and Prevention[2] and PLOS ONE.[3] Trowbridge also published an article in the Culture of Health special edition of *Health Affairs*.[4]

"I had to let go of the way I had been trained and learn to ask questions of architecture friends," said Trowbridge. The team had an "aha moment" when an architect named Dina began to understand the goals of the project, but realized she didn't know how to design it. "This stuff is amazing, but I don't know what to draw," she said. Her comment became somewhat of a mantra, Trowbridge recalled, with the team recognizing that its work would not be finished until "Dina knew what to draw."

Reaching for Scale

Along with going deep in Dillwyn, Trowbridge considers scaling essential to make health a shared value across the built environment field. The green movement is one such strategy, and it is ripe for further scaling. The Green Health Partnership, which has Robert Wood Johnson Foundation (RWJF) support, is a leading vehicle for advancing that movement. A collaborative venture between the University of Virginia and the U.S. Green Building Council, the partnership aims to "create new market interventions that will influence the investment and designs of the built environment sector."

The green movement "writ large has created a very clear cascading value chain all the way from the folks who finance the built environment down to people who have to build and maintain it," noted Trowbridge. Its value chain gives all stakeholders a mandate to think about sustainability and a value proposition that is relevant to their daily work. Close to 80,000 projects have received Leadership in Energy and Environmental (LEED) Design certification from the U.S. Green Building Council, and there are now more than 200,000 certified LEED practitioners.

That kind of system-level transformation has the potential to attract institutional investors at a global level and promote better health across a broad canvas.

But it doesn't happen quickly or easily. "Have some humility about what you know and what you don't know. Really learn what it is that somebody needs to do," said Trowbridge. "Think about Dina, she needs to know what to draw."

Public Life and Human Experience in Public Spaces

In the realm of practice in city-building, we have prioritized everything but people and life . . . even though we build spaces in the service of people
—Shin-pei Tsay

Public life is what happens when people connect in public spaces. Public life encompasses everyday routines, cultural norms, community assets, and social and civic activities that characterize people and the areas they frequent. As such, it shares many components of the social determinants of health.

Gehl Institute aims to transform the way cities are shaped by making people and public life intentional drivers of design, policy, and governance. By measuring the impact of public spaces on the people who use them, the institute seeks to better understand how they contribute to well-being, prosperity, culture, resiliency, and equality.

The institute brings a research and advocacy perspective to the Copenhagen-based Gehl practice, a group of practitioners who work to enhance the human experience in public spaces through evidence-based "people-first" design projects.

A body of evidence highlights features of the environment that create lively spaces, bring people together, and promote active living. Less research has been conducted on the *human experiences* of visiting those spaces, but that is beginning to change. "Coming from the practice side of research and building research from observations in practice, we are now converging in a fundamental way and drawing connections to public health," said Shin-pei Tsay. "We have developed different ways of measuring that, of looking at people in space."

Tsay noted that efforts to change the built environment have traditionally come from the top down. With the devolution of power to the states and less federal leadership in large-scale projects, opportunities are emerging for new models that put the human experience at the center of planning. For example, Gehl Institute's analysis of New York City's Times Square showed that 90 percent of the space was used by cars, yet cars carried only 10 percent of the people trying to navigate that space. Based on that kind of evidence, several blocks in Times Square were converted to pedestrian-only areas, with chairs and benches that allow people to sit, observe, and converse.

The Human Dimension as Starting Point

Along with online research, Gehl Institute uses interviews and observation methods such as counting, mapping, photographing, and conducting test walks to understand how people experience public spaces.

Through this iterative system of study/test/feedback/refine and repeat, Gehl Institute has developed evidence-based tools and metrics that measure people's experiences in public spaces and the relationship between the design of space and socioeconomic factors. For example, a "public life diversity toolkit" identifies where social mixing takes place and the design cues that invite interactions. A "public space, public life survey" counts the number of people using a public space and combines the count with an assessment of the quality, comfort, and safety of the space. "A Mayor's Guide to Public Life" offers strategies, resources, and real-world case studies for mayors.

Learning Block by Block

We really focus on the block level, the people interacting at the block level.
And we dive into the social connections aspects of the research.
—Shin-pei Tsay

To probe the varied nature of social interactions in public spaces, Gehl Institute analyzes passive contacts (merely walking past people), chance contacts (stopping to pet a stranger's dog), "familiar-stranger" contacts (getting to recognize others who frequent the public space), and friendships that develop after repeated encounters. The goal is to understand how contacts build up to create social connections and, ultimately, social cohesion. Their research is "trying to isolate the design elements that instigate or catalyze social space," said Tsay.

A project in Lexington, Kentucky, provides one example. A large landscape development over a broad area of public space was a priority for Lexington officials, but many neighborhoods were not involved in decisions about the space and would not benefit from it. "We had noticed that the parks throughout downtown Lexington did not really have a lot of 'stickiness,'" Tsay said, meaning that people didn't stay long in them.

Based on block-level observation and interview data collected by the institute, Lexington officials installed a SplashJam—an area where children play in water from fountains spouting up from the ground—in an unused plot of land. *That* generated interest. Forty percent of the visitors came from within the surrounding neighborhood, walking to the site and typically staying 30 to 60 minutes. SplashJam became a feature of neighborhood life.

A Strategy Abandoned

While many of its analytical techniques worked well, Gehl had less success when it tried to use social media as a vehicle for determining the popularity of a public space. Although visitors to public spaces posted to social media at high rates, the posts ultimately provided little information about the surrounding neighborhood or social connections among visitors, partly because many who posted were tourists. "We also realized that we did not have the technical capacity to do the required analysis," noted Tsay. Gehl Institute abandoned this study but plans to share the tools it developed so that they can be used by others better positioned to learn from social media.

Reflections on the Pursuit of Scale

A lively and far-reaching discussion followed the presentations, further probing issues of human rights, the built environment, public life in public spaces, and other efforts to scale effective programs. Sanchez opened by noting some of the ingredients that had emerged as necessary to scale effective interventions. Expertise in and understanding of the science of a field is essential, along with a sense of methodology and some rigor around an evaluation. "You also need capital, humility, and a commitment to co-create with others," he said.

Health and Human Rights

JudyAnn Bigby, MD, executive director of South Africa Partners at Harvard Medical School and former senior fellow at Mathematica Policy Research, asked Mariner to elaborate on a statement she had made about health sometimes being "an instrumental good rather than the primary end goal." Since "making health a shared value" is one element of RWJF's Action Framework, Bigby asked, "How can we more explicitly bring the value of health to the forefront of that discussion?"

Mariner elaborated on her point, emphasizing that people have different views about the value of health. For those who do not perceive health as being the primary good that drives actions, it can be valuable to appeal to other goals and framing health as a way to achieve them.

"If one principle is that being healthy and staying healthy is an esteemed social value, what is not being healthy? What are you? Are you shunned?" Mariner asked. She recalled Risa Lavizzo-Mourey's comments at the conference opening: "The choices people make are so often dependent on the choices that they have, and culture is part of the way that we collectively determine the choices people have."

In focusing too much on behavior and not enough on circumstances—the cards people are dealt—we tend to ignore the structures that create the circumstances and place too much blame on the individual. "I don't want to lose the value in the health piece, but I don't want it to be perverted," Mariner said.

Tsay saw reason for optimism in Mariner's perspective. "When I go to different places that have been decimated by economic forces, there are so many leaders, community leaders, who are owning the stewardship of their public spaces. They completely understand the value of what they are bringing," within and beyond the sphere of health.

The Built Environment

Lynne M. Dearborn, PhD, associate professor of architecture, University of Illinois at Urbana-Champaign, observed that the kinds of built environment projects presented in the session face multiple challenges. "Billions of dollars go into design and construction of new environments every year. There is not enough information like they [Trowbridge and Tsay] are showing us for me to give my students when I ask them to design healthy environments. The same resources expended toward new buildings can maintain the status quo or create healthier environments."

The work is not only in the realm of educational environments and public space, but needs to take place in office buildings and elsewhere, Dearborn noted. "I think it's getting in dialogue with designers and planners at the start, as Matthew [Trowbridge] pointed out, learning to bridge the language barriers they encounter and the conceptual barriers that exist."

The challenge goes beyond lack of information, according to Trowbridge. "I don't think right now designers and others who make places have a mandate to incorporate health into their plans. When you go deep, you see what happens when there is a mandate."

To amplify his point, Trowbridge described a green charrette exploring housing in San Francisco (charrettes are structured, intense discussions among stakeholders, often architects, charged with developing solutions within a deadline). "They had the architects, sure, but they also had all the structural engineers, the water engineers, and the city finance people," he observed. "There were solution providers everywhere, and the goal that day was to set the sustainability goals for the project."

Trowbridge also observed that the charrette was not mandated to consider health within the housing project. That experience led him to three questions: Why can't ordinances require a health charrette? Why don't we have health solution providers, just as we have green solution providers? And why are educators not training master's in public health students interested in the built environment to "go out and be practical, to be solution providers"?

One possible course of action for architects:

> *I am a licensed architect, and that license says I am responsible for the health, safety, and welfare of everyone using the spaces I design. This is a call to our National Council of Architectural Registration Boards that this does not mean only the building codes. It is broader than that.*
> *—Audience Member*

Role of Government

One audience member questioned whether public agencies other than extremely large ones, such as the Centers for Medicare and Medicaid Services, would commit to funding large-scale evidence-based programs. Noting that large-scale prevention initiatives are expensive, another participant asked whether there was any hope for implementing them without players willing to absorb their cost.

Nirav Shah, director on the social investment team of Social Finance, agreed that while many government agencies want to invest in prevention programs, fiscal, structural, and political barriers often thwart their efforts, especially those likely to yield benefits only years after the costs have been incurred. "I think there are pockets of opportunities, but it's rare," he said.

Referencing South Carolina's Pay for Success financing model, which braids Medicaid funds with private investments (for more on Pay for Success, see Chapter 7, "Making the Economic Case for Population Health"), Nirav Shah said, "The project allows South Carolina to scale an evidence-based prevention program while providing a pathway for the state to sustain the services with Medicaid funding if the project generates positive results."

That's an example of stakeholders thinking more broadly about return on investments, he continued. "The best example I have is infant mortality. How do you put a price on reducing infant mortality?" Nirav Shah also observed that a fundamental role of government is to improve lives and promote equal opportunity, principles that go beyond finance.

Legal/Moral Obligations and Financial Impact

Seth A. Berkowitz, MD, MPH, a researcher at Massachusetts General Hospital, commented that divergent visions were being put forward for developing policies that shape social determinants of health. One vision advances a legal and perhaps moral obligation to make change, while the other emphasizes financing. "It seemed like those are divergent justifications, and I would like to hear more about reconciling them," he said.

Elaborating on the issue, Berkowitz added, "If I'm trying to come up with a new cancer treatment, I would establish efficacy and we would figure out the financing later on. But for a lot of social determinants, it seems like people are saying not only does it need to improve social outcomes, but it has to be done at an acceptable cost."

Trowbridge pointed to two factors that can influence thinking here. First, when the green movement was new, architects and investors involved in green building gained a reputation for being high performers. "The green movement has become so standardized and so normative that it's boring, which is awesome," he commented. Acceptance of green construction has created an opportunity for stakeholders to demonstrate that there is a process for intentionally addressing health in all aspects of development. "That is the new differentiator, that makes you high performance," he said.

> There is a really cool opportunity to push people to be more aggressive, telling them, "If you build this now, I swear ten years from now, you are going to regret that you did not have an intentional health strategy."
> —Matthew Trowbridge

Risk reduction is the second factor offering hope for progress and for integrating moral and financial visions. A building lasts for years, so if something is missed that could have helped to generate health, that gap remains for a long time.

A Final Word

A society marked by equity and well-being rests on effective, robust interventions that have both deep roots and broad reach. Policies that attack structural and environmental problems at their core provide a foundation for the interaction between knowledge and action and create the context for addressing the social determinants that undermine a Culture of Health.

Political tensions at the national level, coupled with a growing tendency to turn decision-making back to the states, create new pressures and new opportunities for community and state leadership to bring about social change. Fortunately, neither the challenges nor the solutions are the domain of the United States alone. As suggested by the involvement of the Gehl Institute, with its roots in Denmark, and the international human rights frame offered in this chapter, there is a global context for state and local initiatives to test and scale ideas.

13

Bridging the Academia–Media Gap

AL CROSS

Director, Institute for Rural Journalism and Community Issues, University of Kentucky

LISA SIMPSON, MB, BCH, MPH, FAAP

President and Chief Executive Officer, Academy Health

News media, including local newspapers rooted in their towns or regions, play a critical role in translating evidence for policymakers, practitioners, and the public. By telling meaningful stories, journalists make clear the fiscal, political, and human implications of policy options. By putting scientific information into the public domain, they promote the free exchange of the grounded ideas that are essential to productive discussions about issues of broad concern.

Today, researchers and journalists alike are working in uncertain environments characterized by rapidly changing expectations and norms. Although publication in peer-reviewed journals is still an essential goal of research and critical to generating knowledge, its contribution to problem-solving is increasingly perceived as limited unless it also contributes to public discourse. Yet many researchers are not trained to think about the policy implications of their work and often find it difficult to frame their studies that way.

At the same time, publishers have less money to hire specialist reporters, increasingly relying instead on generalists to cover a range of topics. Editors may base story selection more on a desire for a larger audience than on educating that audience. Reporters face tighter deadlines, have less space in which to develop a story, and are edited less vigorously.

Changes in technology have also significantly affected both professions. Increased access to publicly available data, for example, enables researchers to demonstrate how a big-picture finding about a national trend is experienced by people living in a town of interest to a local reporter. The same access also gives journalists opportunities to analyze the data and draw their own conclusions.

The contributors to this chapter—one immersed in the world of research and one a journalist—offer perspectives on the academia–media gap and explore ways to bridge it.

The Research Perspective

Through a program of conferences, scholarships and fellowships, and partnerships between researchers and policymakers, AcademyHealth supports the productive use of evidence to inform health policy and practice. Lisa Simpson opened this session with observations on the role of research within the policy arena.

A robust and dynamic news media is a cornerstone of a democratic society, she said. Research contributes to media coverage by informing public discourse and providing evidence about policy challenges and failures, supporting media outlets in their essential watchdog function.

Publishing in peer-reviewed scientific journals remains essential to vet the quality of a study, as well as to advance a researcher's career. But the emphasis on technical language and research methodology means that most journal articles do not readily translate into principles that can be applied to real-world settings. To draw wider coverage of their work in popular media, Simpson urged researchers to be relevant, honest, and authentic; quotable and interesting; reliable; and timely.

She also described some of the efforts being made to document the connections between research and media. The use of altmetrics[1]—metrics and qualitative data that complement citation-based metrics to track popular coverage of research findings—represents one effort to measure the reach of research findings beyond scientific journals. The *Journal of the American Medical Association*, for example, uses altmetrics to track mentions of articles on Twitter and blogs and in popular media.

In addition to getting their information from colleagues, Beltway publications, and the Congressional Research Service, policymakers turn to

- The Internet, a source for 89 percent of policymakers
- The national press, a source for 84 percent of policymakers
- Academic and issue experts, a source for 73 percent of policymakers

Language and Context

Some words and phrases provoke emotional responses or favor one political belief over another, said Simpson. In the current polarized environment, in which people interpret new information as confirmation of their opinions—called *confirmation bias*—framing evidence thoughtfully and choosing language carefully are important to promoting civic dialogue.

For example, "public health" tends to evoke a different response than "nanny state." This is not to suggest that inaccurate or intentionally misleading terms should ever be used, but only to highlight the way language affects how an audience receives a message and to encourage conscious choice in framing hot-button issues.

In addition, findings that are placed within the context of a larger body of evidence are likely to be more useful to policymakers than a single finding or study and of greater interest to reporters. If they can readily understand how one study compares with other evidence about the topic or adds new perspective to it, reporters are more likely to cover it.

> *Researchers can make their studies compelling by learning how to frame their findings using language that convinces reporters they should care about the findings.*
> —Lisa Simpson

Speeding Up Dissemination

The standard research trajectory—conducting the study, publishing findings in a scientific journal, and then perhaps having them covered in a popular media outlet—is out of sync with the needs of policymakers and the general public, who often must make decisions quickly, whether or not they have solid evidence to support them.

The advent of online publication has shortened the time between completing a study and publishing its findings, but publication often remains a lengthy process. As a result, many researchers have turned to more timely dissemination strategies, including policy briefs, blogs, and open-access journals. Evidence reviews, which provide policymakers with an overview of a body of evidence rather than findings from a single study, can be developed more quickly, but their validity has not been established. With support from Robert Wood Johnson Foundation, staff at AcademyHealth is reviewing the conclusions reached by evidence reviews of various policy strategies. "What do evidence summaries find if they are produced in two days, two weeks, or six weeks?" said Simpson.

Cultivating Relationships

Researchers do well to think about media and dissemination as they launch their studies and to anticipate tough questions from the start. When preparing for meetings with media representatives, Simpson asks, "What is the question I absolutely do not want to answer?"—and then decides how she will handle that question.

She advised researchers to reach out to journalists. Even if journalists do not need information at the time, building relationships promotes trust and sets the stage for future engagement. It also gives researchers opportunities to educate journalists about a topic.

People like to read stories about their communities or regions. When researchers relate national data to local developments, a journalist can show local readers and residents why they are relevant. "That generates attention," said Simpson. Reflecting on many of the conference presentations, Simpson concludes, "Your data make you credible. And your stories make you memorable."

The Media Perspective

As director of the Institute for Rural Journalism and Community Issues at the University of Kentucky, Al Cross helps rural journalists "define the public agenda for their communities and grasp the local impact of broader issues." Rural journalism is important because 16 percent of Americans— 63 million people—live in rural areas, and 75 percent of the American landscape is rural.

Cross emphasized that while reporters disseminate findings from research, they are not performing a public relations function and prefer not to get most of their information from an institution's public relations staff. "We want to talk to the real sources, the researchers themselves," Cross said. Newspapers want fresh copy, and few are just going to post an institution's press release on their sites.

A reporter is paid to ask tough questions, to practice a discipline of verification.
—Al Cross

If a reporter and editor do decide to cover a story, Cross said, "They are standing for the information in that story. And they have a First Amendment obligation to examine every angle." That is better accomplished through direct discussions between the researcher and the reporter.

Still, after 26 years as a reporter for the *Courier-Journal* of Louisville, Cross understands the challenges in covering the health agenda. "I avoided health care stories like the plague," he admitted. "It was too much, too arcane, too complicated, and too easy to make a mistake."

National Stories, Local Angles

Researchers seeking coverage in popular media outlets have to capture the interest of the reporter, their first audience. To do that, Cross recommended boiling down a key provocative finding to a headline, "Think of a tweet," he suggested. "Try to fit your point into 140 characters."

Stories are also more likely to be printed—and read—if they are selective about what they promote and are pitched to the primary interests of each intended audience. Cross urged researchers to consider whether they are targeting policymakers or the general public.

A local focus is often paramount because most newspapers in the United States emphasize local news so that they do not compete with larger papers. Surveys show that readers trust their local newspapers more than they trust metropolitan papers or national news media. Since local papers generally come out weekly, they are likely to remain in homes for the full week and residents may refer to them more than once.

Studies that feature both national trends and local data appeal to "relentlessly local" newspapers. Many of them welcome opportunities to show how a trend in the country as a whole affects local readers, listeners, and viewers. In assembling the institute's *The Rural Blog*, "we look for things that have local resonance," said Cross.

He presented excerpts drawn from national studies that were published in *The Rural Blog* and commented about their relevance to local audiences:

- "Study says surgeries are safer and cheaper at critical-access hospitals, which are rural." (Cross: "Rural hospitals are a huge concern to my clientele.")
- "Cancer deaths on the rise in parts of the South and Appalachia, despite overall decline, study finds." (Cross: "We love research that involves county-by-county data.")

He also offered an example of how such studies can make powerful stories for local newspapers:

- "Hickman County: What's Killing Us" (A headline about the county's leading causes of death from the *Hickman County Times* of Centerville, Tennessee)

A Bias for Good News

There is a "cheerleader mentality" in community newspapers, a mentality Cross' institute is trying to change. The better local papers hold up a mirror to their community, prodding leaders to face and address unflattering conditions. More often, however, papers hesitate to publish stories that reflect poorly on their community. When researchers at the University of Kentucky tailored findings about individual counties to those counties, based on *County Health Rankings & Roadmaps*, few of the county papers ran a story about them.

"The lower your health ranking in Kentucky, the less likely you are to read about it in your local newspaper, and the better your health ranking, the more likely you are to read about it," Cross noted. Many papers were more likely to run "advertorials, or advertisements masquerading as news" than research findings that are uncomplimentary, he said.

There are indications that this is changing, however. The institute's 2015 and 2017 analyses of the *County Health Rankings & Roadmaps* coverage of Kentucky found no discernible difference between healthier and unhealthier counties, according to Cross. In addition, the number of stories increased in 2017, with more than 25 percent of counties featuring stories that year.

Emerging Media Outlets: New Opportunities

Traditional newspapers and television outlets have cut back on staff dedicated to health and on the column space and air time they dedicate to health stories. While many papers increasingly do publish special sections on health, these sections are sometimes heavy with advertorial or other paid content.

Online news outlets, on the other hand, are launching in communities across the country and they "are hungry for copy," said Cross. "Don't ignore the online outlets as good places for getting stuff out," he urged.

The institute's *Kentucky Health News*, an online journal, features events and trends about health care and health in Kentucky. Georgia, North Carolina, and other states have developed similar online outlets. "*Kentucky Health News* tries to make news people can use, based on research," Cross said. "We are not aimed at policymakers. We limit our items to research that has impact on readers."

> I think that even though newspaper readership is down, newspapers are still the most-read source of information and the greatest source of in-depth information.
> —Al Cross

Print newspapers often lift stories from *Kentucky Health News* and publish them as news articles, expanding their reach. "We have been encouraged by the growth in health news coverage in Kentucky newspapers since this project started, and we'd like to think that we have had something to do with it," Cross said. "Several newspapers run something from us every week, and have created a regular page for health news, [and] most of the stories on these pages are ours. Likewise, more papers are doing special health sections, and we provide a lot of copy for those."

Reflections on a Complex Relationship

Simpson engaged Cross and audience participants in a conversation to dig deeper into trends of interest. "Data journalism" is one such trend. Increased access to data, combined with easy-to-use online graphics programs, puts new tools in the hands of journalists. In "data journalism, journalists do their own research," Cross said. "They get publicly available data and they write stories." (For more on the opportunities and challenges that arise from the increasing availability of data, see Chapter 9, "Traditional and New Data: Competing or Compatible?")

Another trend, and one of concern, is greater sensationalism and less attention to caveats, limitations, and qualifiers. Cross recalls hearing one newspaper editor say that the essential element of journalism is that it should be interesting, without mentioning the importance of truth, accuracy, fairness, independence, or relevance. "That shows how hungry newspapers are for audience," he observed.

Turning to social media, Simpson noted that researchers have not been major users of Twitter, Facebook, or new platforms, embracing them more slowly than people in other fields. That pattern, however, is changing as social media becomes an increasingly powerful and pervasive presence across disciplines, sectors, and professions.

"Social media now rule the day, and researchers have to be there," Cross agreed. Every post on *The Rural Blog* and on *Kentucky Health News* generates a tweet. The biggest pitfall, Cross said, is "getting sucked into a thread of commentary that lacks the discipline of verification," an essential element of journalism.

Short (60- to 90-second) videos posted on Twitter or other social media platforms are an untapped resource for researchers. Funding the development of best practices for using short videos in social media outlets would be money well spent, Cross observed. A video can highlight key points and refer viewers to a more complete body of research, but "you have to get their attention first."

Niels Lund, MSc, MBA, vice president of health advocacy at Novo Nordisk, asked whether researchers would be better served by reaching out directly to policymakers, rather than by engaging with journalists. Informing policy, Lund asserted, requires dialogue that might be more productive without media involvement.

In some circumstances, researchers should work directly with policymakers, Cross agreed. But he cautioned that often, "you will find only a few people who are willing to go to bat for you and carry the ball." Politicians are responsive to constituents, and the best way to reach constituents with this kind of message is through media, he said.

Simpson cited an early study of deaths due to hospital error as a case in point. "We [researchers] had the data and we had the information, but not until the Institute of Medicine published *To Err Is Human* [1999], and put a number to the deaths, did anything happen." Her take-away: researchers who generate findings before policymakers are interested in them should be ready, "so when the time is right, you can throw findings into the conversation."

Randall Brown, PhD, director of health research senior fellows at Mathematica Policy Research, sparked a conversation about the difficulties that arise when, as Cross recommended, researchers try to sidestep their institutions' press offices and speak directly to journalists. Federal research contracts include rules requiring researchers to work through the agency's press office, and talking directly to a reporter can get them in real trouble, Brown said.

After an initial interview involving the press office, researchers may be able to respond directly if reporters call with follow-up questions. In any conversation, take time to offer a considered answer, urged Cross. "Don't feel like you're compelled to give an answer right then." Asking for time to respond is accepted practice, as long as researchers know journalists' deadlines and respect them.

Brown's concern raises larger issues of intellectual independence, freedom to publish, and freedom to speak. Speaking to the media is just one dimension of this independence, said Simpson. Another involves restrictions applied by funders of the work itself. For example, federal agencies are increasingly funding research through contracts rather than grants, which can impose more restrictions on researcher independence.

Several participants expressed opinions about incorporating a human angle in stories, a common journalistic technique. Reporters often want a human face—a patient, physician, or clinic administrator who can talk about a situation. Because that requires a trusted partner willing to offer a personal perspective, Simpson recommended that researchers raise the topic early in their studies, asking key people interested in the implications of a study whether they would be willing to be interviewed if the media wants to cover it.

Some audience members were uncomfortable with stories that turn to senior officials for a human angle because readers or viewers may view their perspective with suspicion. Cross shared that concern, suggesting that editors of local publications may have more credibility with readers. Rural readers and editors "think of themselves as community newspaper people or local television people," he said. "They care about a locality and sometimes they worry that experts do not understand rural or remote areas. If people trust their local editors, that communicates instant credibility."

John Moon, MPP, district manager of community development at the Federal Reserve Bank of San Francisco, raised the idea of linking topics not generally associated with health, such as housing and transportation, to health policies. Demonstrating the health effects of nonhealth policies, such as those that drive gentrification, might spark interest among journalists, he thought.

Cross agreed that a "health in all policies" strategy, one that brings a health question to a debate about other topics, might better leverage reporters' interests because it broadens the audience interested in those questions.

One participant recalled conducting a literature review in which she realized that newspapers are a good source of process information, day-to-day decisions, and stories about how things happen. Cross agreed, citing an adage often attributed to former *Washington Post* president and publisher Philip L. Graham: "Journalism is the first rough draft of history." At least some of what journalists write now will be read by someone else decades later.

A Final Word

Today, more than ever, evidence needs to be unassailable and communicated clearly, simply, and accurately. Heated discussion in the media about what constitutes "facts" points to the low level of trust people now place in research and evidence, making it essential that research conclusions are rigorous and cannot be challenged on the basis of their accuracy.

Researchers can contribute to a Culture of Health by exploring what promotes or inhibits personal and societal well-being. Their findings shine a light on trends, promising practices, and unaddressed problems. Journalists do their part by then framing that evidence in terms of policy options and lived experiences in communities. Together, the work can catalyze action. In bridging the academia–media gap, researchers and journalists together set the stage for informed debate, better policies, and stronger programs.

14

Failing Forward

Pitfalls and Progress

VERONICA COMBS

Executive Director, Institute for Healthy Air, Water, and Soil

LENA HATCHETT, PHD

Assistant Professor and Director of Community and University Partnerships,
Loyola University Chicago

GABRIEL LARA

Executive Director, Quinn Community Center

ROHIT RAMASWAMY, PHD, MPH

Associate Professor, Public Health Leadership Program; Director for Global Learning Gillings
School of Global Public Health, University of North Carolina at Chapel Hill

SAMUEL ROSS, MD, MS

Chief Executive Officer, Bon Secours Baltimore Health System; Executive Vice President,
Bon Secours Health System, Inc.

> *If you don't get paralyzed by failing, you rethink ways of working and you*
> *listen. And that, I think, is beautiful.*
>
> —*Gabriel Lara*

"Failing forward" is a philosophy and a strategy of learning from mistakes that has made its way into the popular lexicon over the past decade. It starts with acknowledging, sometimes publicly, that an idea did not work. People who fail forward strive to understand what went wrong—and then they try again, usually with a different approach. The hope is that by transforming their mistakes into knowledge and insights, they become more steadfast, bold, and creative. In failing forward, they seek better outcomes for their organizations and often find meaningful personal growth through the experience, allowing them to become more thoughtful, effective citizens.

The four contributors to this chapter tell their personal stories of failing forward, describing well-intentioned but initially ill-fated efforts to bring about change in their communities. In working to improve air quality in Louisville; engage with evaluators in Maywood, Illinois; provide free food to residents of Maywood; and manage a health coalition in Baltimore, they demonstrate the wherewithal to acknowledge their mistakes without becoming incapacitated by them.

Rohit Ramaswamy moderated the session, asking "what does it take" not to be afraid to make mistakes. He engaged with contributors and audience members in lessons-learned conversations following each presentation and facilitated a broader exploration of cross-cutting themes at the end of the workshop.

Improving Air Quality in Louisville

In Louisville, asthma is the number-one reason children end up in emergency departments, and it is a significant cause of absenteeism from school and work. As executive director of the Institute for Healthy Air, Water, and Soil, a nonprofit agency formed in 2014, Veronica Combs wanted to change that picture.

The institute launched with fanfare, sponsoring a public event to promote the purchase and use of "air quality eggs"—attractive egg-shaped sensors people hang in their yards to monitor air quality and pollution around their homes. The idea behind the eggs was to empower residents by giving them real-time information about the air in their immediate environment. "The eggs were cute and had a catchy name," said Combs, recalling the launch as a great event that generated some press coverage.

But the excitement was short-lived as the eggs soon created more problems than they solved. The sensors were excessively responsive, reporting air quality problems when none existed. "People understandably started freaking out," Combs said. Forced to backtrack, the institute retrieved the air quality eggs and eased people's fears about breathing bad air. Combs realized the eggs "were not ready for prime time."

The institute regrouped—it failed forward—seeking other strategies to give residents real-time information about the air they breathed. Using data collected by the federal Environmental Protection Agency from sensors scattered around Louisville, the institute developed a system for sending air quality alerts to residents based on data recorded by the sensors located nearest to their homes. In the process, it forged enduring partnerships with city officials and residents, generating a higher level of interest in air quality that has paid off in the long run.

The institute's failing forward experience has shown results, but much work remains to be done to improve air quality in Louisville. For example, the Environmental Protection Agency sensors often go offline, and because they record air quality over an eight-hour period, they mask air quality spikes that occur during the course of a day. Louisville's location, separated from the state of Indiana only by the Ohio River, poses another challenge. Its residents are affected by the air quality in Indiana but have no authority over regulations in that state.

While the air quality eggs are no longer part of Louisville's strategy, "People still ask us about the eggs," said Combs. "And I say, 'Well, we have moved on.'"

Lessons Learned

As a small nonprofit, the institute had more flexibility than larger city agencies to implement the air quality egg program and then to abandon it quickly when problems arose. It did not have to navigate cumbersome bureaucracies when things started to go wrong or to confront a political environment that attributes failures to waste or incompetence.

Other lessons emerged as well. The decision to use Environmental Protection Agency data allowed the institute to base its work on neutral information, which made it easier for the institute to convene people with diverse and sometimes conflicting views about pollution. Having multiple air quality projects under way helped the institute keep the community focused on air quality. A grant from the Robert Wood Johnson Foundation (RWJF), for example, allowed it to purchase sensors that attach to an asthma inhaler. The sensors send notices to a smartphone whenever the inhaler is used, creating a record of asthma attacks over time.

Sometimes, residents in low-income areas indicate they do not want their air quality recorded, noted a few members of the audience. Being labeled as having bad air, some residents believed, contributes to perceptions that the neighborhood is undesirable, has high crime rates, and suffers from other social problems—or low-income residents may work for companies that pollute the air and do not want their employers to come under scrutiny for contributing to pollution.

Even though it did not ultimately work, addressing these concerns had been one of the compelling aspects of the air quality eggs, said Combs. "One of the reasons we wanted people to have their own egg was to let them see their own data and draw their own conclusions." They could then take whatever action they felt appropriate. "We really did not want to get in the role of being pigeonholed as any particular kind of political institution," she added.

Combs's biggest lesson from the air quality egg experience: "I learned that you have to persist, you have to show the value of failure."

Overcoming Personal and Professional Insecurity in Maywood, Illinois

Proviso Partners for Health is a multisector coalition that supports community health and promotes health equity in and around Maywood, a suburb of Chicago, Illinois. Residents of these towns face high rates of obesity and unemployment, struggling schools, and limited transportation services. "Too many people see no clear opportunities out of that situation," said Lena Hatchett, Proviso's executive director.

Proviso began in 2014 as a loose association of just three organizations trying to bring healthy food choices to Maywood. Three years later, Proviso includes more than 35 public and nonprofit partners dedicated to developing a sustainable food system in which young people prepare and distribute healthy, affordable food. Profits from food sales return to the community.

As Proviso Partners for Health grew, Hatchett found herself in new professional territory, at times facing issues and decisions outside her experience and level of comfort. She did not want "to tell people how much I did not know, and I certainly didn't want to tell our funders and our community how unprepared we were for [addressing] large-scale community health."

The pressure to evaluate Proviso's community health initiatives elevated these concerns, prompting Hatchett's transformative failing forward experience. "I knew if we could solve the problem of community-wide evaluation, we could go to scale," she said, but she was not at first ready to admit she lacked the expertise to guide such an endeavor.

The stakes for Hatchett were high. Residents were understandably skittish about engaging with outside evaluators who often enter their communities with a focus on rigid numeric outcomes at the expense of measuring factors of local importance, such as neighborhood context and assets. At the same time, Hatchett believed that results from an evaluation would strengthen community capacity, help local businesses maximize profit, and reassure residents that the food system was producing reliable sources of healthy food at reasonable prices.

Hatchett credits her participation in RWJF's Spreading Community Accelerators through Learning and Evaluation (SCALE) program with enabling her to break through her fears—to fail forward. Through SCALE-sponsored training and technical assistance, she became more aware of and comfortable with her unique role as convener and guide.

With that insight, Hatchett started bringing evaluators and residents together, ensuring that the evaluation would work for both. As her confidence grew, she more readily asked evaluators for explanations when she didn't understand a point. The more she asked, the more she and Proviso's partners learned about community-wide evaluations.

Lessons Learned

The discussion about the lessons learned from Hatchett's experience focused on building community–evaluator relationships with neighborhood residents who organized into an evaluation team of community improvement advisers. One measure of importance to community members is identifying their assets and opportunities, good places to begin addressing problems collaboratively.

> *The thing we learned by failing forward is that while it was a challenge to go back over our failing moments, that was the exact place we needed to start in order to succeed.*
> —Lena Hatchett

Making the point that "what gets measured is what becomes important," an audience member asked which assets Proviso's community residents chose to be measured through the evaluation. "Community self-esteem," Hatchett said. "We are measuring the concept of community self-esteem and capacity building."

Somava (Soma) Stout, MD, MS, vice president at the Institute of Healthcare Improvement (which directs SCALE), noted that evaluations that focus on whether something succeeded or did not succeed can damage community interventions trying to tackle complex problems. She reported that Proviso Partners for Health has "some of the best outcomes in all of SCALE, and the kinds of outcomes it has been able to pursue—economic development, healthy food consumption, or growth in leadership capacity—are far more interesting than outcomes they might have started out to explore. It wasn't until they were a quarter of the way in that they figured out what measures would actually matter. If they were evaluated only on what they started with, we would have missed the whole picture."

Hatchett's take-away lesson from failing forward is her realization that while she did not speak the language of evaluation, she had a clear vision for what the evaluation should do, and the community had that vision as well. Her role was to promote a healthy and equal partnership between the evaluators and community members.

Rethinking the Meaning of Charity in Maywood, Illinois

St. Eulalia Catholic Church in Maywood has a history of providing services to people in need, no questions asked. The church's commitment to charity, justice, peace, and equity have undergirded its philosophy that aid should be offered without asking anything from the people receiving it.

Gabriel Lara, executive director of St. Eulalia's Quinn Community Center, recounted the church's failing forward experience, which took years to unfold.

Since the day St. Eulalia opened its food pantry in 1970, volunteers have provided free food to everyone who needed it. By about 2000, however, food resources had dwindled and fewer people were visiting the pantry. Church leaders did not know why and, upon reflection, recognized that the church's no-questions-asked philosophy of charitable giving had prevented it from developing deep ties to the community. "We realized that the same people had been coming to the pantry for 20 or 30 years, but nobody but the director of the food pantry knew their names," said Lara.

We didn't know we were failing because we weren't measuring anything.
—Gabriel Lara

Church leaders felt "guilty and ashamed," recalled Lara. Renewing their commitment to church principles, they failed forward, establishing Quinn Community Center to help the church become a good partner with and key resource for Maywood residents. As a first step, St. Eulalia's pastor hired Lara, initially for 10 hours per week, to start asking the questions the church had traditionally been hesitant to ask.

Lara started by talking with food pantry visitors about the circumstances that brought them in and, importantly, about what they would like from the church. "The answers were beautiful," he said. People told him they wanted to be more active partners with the church and to contribute to its services. They also wanted the church to create programs that would allow them to improve their lives so they would no longer need free food.

Lara described his discussions with visitors to the church as the beginning of an informal evaluation. St. Eulalia joined Hatchett's Proviso Partners for Health, and through that connection, Lara learned more about failing forward and tools of collaboration.

Changes followed shortly. After hearing seven women describe their dreams of forming a restaurant, Quinn Community Center offered them classes in health, sanitation, and food preparation. "There are now 30 women who own their own catering enterprise, providing healthy catered food to paying customers," reported Lara.

Working initially with seven young people who received food from the pantry, St. Eulalia now oversees 35 youth who operate a summer program for the church. A church-led collaboration of teachers, parents, and the Chicago-based Golden Apple Foundation provided training and support for the project.

> *We first failed to engage community residents as partners, but when we failed forward we realized we could reach out to them and say, "We are in this together."*
> —*Gabriel Lara*

Lessons Learned

Lara's story sparked a discussion about lessons learned from the feelings of guilt and shame church officials experienced when they realized they didn't know the people who had been visiting the pantry for years. Failing forward can be powerful and effective, no matter when it happens. "It is never too late to fail, as long as it is failing forward," said Lara.

Denise E. Herrera, PhD, a program officer at RWJF, was struck by how the church "took a time out and said, 'We need to listen to our community.'" She asked for suggestions as to how funders, evaluators, and practitioners can become better listeners and view community residents through a culturally responsive lens.

Reflecting on his early conversations with food pantry visitors, Lara said it was important for him to learn "who is that person in front of me, what questions has this person not been asked, what questions will help me understand the richness." Measuring with numbers can overlook the strengths of a person or a community because, in relying on numbers, "we haven't listened," he concluded.

Creating a Health Coalition in Baltimore

Bon Secours Baltimore Health System began providing home health care and other community-based services soon after it was established by the Sisters of Bon Secours in 1881. In 2017, it offers clinical and behavioral health care services and a range of social, employment, early childhood, and prisoner reentry programs through its community outreach component. The health system also operates 700 low-income housing units in West Baltimore.

When he moved to Bon Secours from Dallas's Parkland Health and Hospital System in 2006, Samuel Ross brought with him a commitment to the four components of the community-oriented primary care program: identify the community, listen to residents and learn what is important to them, introduce appropriate interventions, and measure the outcomes. The big question for Ross is, "Did what we said would make a difference actually make a difference?"

Residents of West Baltimore had concerns that went beyond the doors of the hospital and even beyond the purview of the health care system. They told us that "their biggest health problems are the rats and the trash, not hypertension, heart disease, or diabetes, conditions statistics would report as health problems," said Ross.

While impressed with the range of community services offered by the hospital, Ross concluded that it had too often acted on its own. He believed that the future of Bon Secours hinged on its ability to join with other stakeholders in forging a shared vision for the community. A state senator agreed and supported Bon Secours in forming the West Baltimore Primary Care Access Collaborative. The collaborative includes three federally qualified health centers, five hospitals, three community-based organizations, three academic institutions, and city and state policymakers.

"We started having meetings, and people felt good about meeting," Ross recalled with some humor. But the meetings were failing to lead to tangible and important actions. In a collaborative filled with high-powered leaders, "power is not easily ceded," he learned. "Everybody was jockeying to remain at the top."

Faced with an unwieldy collaborative, Ross decided to fail forward—as an individual and on behalf of the collaborative. He convinced stakeholders to spend $100,000 to engage a consultant from the Maryland Conflict Resolution Center to facilitate the meetings. With guidance from the facilitator, the collaborative developed communications protocols, operational procedures, and standards of accountability. When necessary, the facilitator spoke informally and off-the-record to a member, resolving problems quietly and out of the public view. The facilitator "was worth every penny," said Ross.

Ross had a second opportunity to fail forward when a 2013 Health Enterprise Zone grant from the state of Maryland put pressure on the collaborative to reach specified and challenging targets to reduce disparities, costs, and hospital admissions and to improve access to care (for more about Maryland's Health Enterprise Zones, see Chapter 7, "Making the Economic Case for Population Health").

At the end of the first year of the four-year grant, state officials told Ross the collaborative was not meeting its targets and had to refocus its efforts. Changes in leadership at the state level and high turnover among collaborative directors (it has had five executive directors in four years) complicated the problem.

Again, Ross guided the collaborative in failing forward, this time to relinquish control of some programs and contract with community-based organizations to deliver key outreach and coordination services. "We quickly figured out that was the better way, given the limited time we had," he said.

Overcoming these stumbles proved to be milestones for the collaborative, according to Ross: "We have done a lot to pull people together who had not worked together well in the past. We have overcome a lot of the earlier barriers and are now moving more smoothly in the way we hoped."

Reflections on Failing Forward

Audience members engaged with Ramaswamy, contributors, and one another in mining the failing forward experiences for broad themes.

Involve and Empower Community Residents

Dwayne Proctor, PhD, RWJF director and senior adviser to the president, noted that the failing forward experiences were prompted by well-intended but unsuccessful efforts to meaningfully engage community residents and to share authority and control. "My take-away from the presentations is that the idea of bringing people along from the very beginning is a must-do—it has to happen," he said.

Ross replied that the ongoing challenge, and imperative, is helping residents get involved beyond a single program or initiative. Part of the failing forward work at Bon Secours, he said, was preparing community members to play important roles in larger contexts, such as advocating before the city council or other policy venues.

Louisville's Veronica Combs noted the logistical challenges, such as child care and transportation, which often confront low-income residents. "We get paid to do this, but other people are volunteering their time," she reminded the audience.

To build strong and equal partnerships between evaluators and residents, Hatchett asserts, evaluations have to be collaborative and they have to capture measures that are important to residents as well as to the evaluators. She tells evaluators, "Our youth and our seniors are more invested in the evaluation than you are. They live here and they want to see and know the impact more than you do."

The question arose as to whether there are situations in which "the community" is impossible to define. Those working to reduce infant mortality, for example, may find there is not an identifiable community of women at risk for losing children. Ross agreed that identifying the community of interest is not always easy. Hospitals and health systems are built on a "one-size-fits-all" model, he believes, and are not equipped to cope with multiple interactions or to engage in work that involves a lot of listening. However, some audience members challenged the notion that communities cannot be identified, and offered personal examples of stakeholders organizing to speak for themselves.

Bring Health Systems to the Table

Proviso Partners for Health emerged from within the Maywood community, giving Hatchett an alternative perspective on the engagement challenge. "What we need to do is figure out how to engage the health system in community social change, not how to get the community to the table. To make a partnership work, the health sector needs to learn the community context, the community language, and the community priorities."

Exercise Humility

Dennis P. Andrulis, PhD, MPH, senior research scientist at the Texas Health Institute, observed that, in describing their failing forward experiences, contributors demonstrated humility about their work and their constituents. Their capacity to open up about what they did not know and to learn from others was an important factor in successfully failing forward.

Combs offered a case in point. Louisville's Institute for Air, Water, and Soil Quality wanted to "green-up" a neighborhood and then test the impact on the heart health of residents. Then, she recalled, "The institute showed up, asking people, 'Can we plant a tree in your yard? That will help your health.'" Residents, however, were more concerned with crime, afterschool activities, and falling home prices than they were about living in a green environment. The institute recognized it had to do more to address those priorities, as well as its own interests, and to get involved with other local revitalization efforts.

Look Beyond Grants to Sustain an Initiative

Hatchett's work began with community passion but not many other resources. "These are people's lives, and when we are moving toward a Culture of Health, that is not a project, it is not a grant. Those things are not the foundation of our sustainability."

From Hatchett's perspective, sustainability has to emerge from the activities that community residents take to improve people's lives. For example, food sales from Proviso-created businesses generate revenue, with profits reinvested in the community. "I would urge everyone to think about sustainability early and not rely on grant funds, especially in this climate," she concluded.

Respect Service as Highly as Research

Hatchett observed that although she had been doing community-based participatory research throughout her career, "It is my community-based participatory service that got me here today, not the research." Research is important, but it takes research, services, *and* community organizing to create the social change needed for a Culture of Health, she said.

A Final Word

In real life, things go wrong, and implementing programs on the ground often really is "rocket science." Community residents struggle every day to address significant social determinants of health without adequate resources, sufficient time, technical expertise, or political leverage, often in the face of conflicting opinions about the best course of action. Researchers and residents have yet to learn how to fully engage with one another in community settings.

The challenges are daunting, but the potential is real and powerful. The personal stories told here bring to life many of the challenges of community engagement and collaboration that have been described elsewhere in this book. They also illuminate pathways to better outcomes. Failing forward happens in organizations as dissimilar as a small food pantry in suburban Illinois and a large hospital system in Baltimore. The lessons that emerge apply as much to Louisville, Kentucky, as they do to Maywood, Illinois.

By guiding their agencies in failing forward, Combs, Hatchett, Lara, and Ross modeled deep commitment to community, determined intelligence that resists easy answers, and enough self-assurance to admit their mistakes. In failing forward, they rejected blame, anger, and despair and chose instead collaboration, reflection, and determination.

SECTION V

PROFILES OF KENTUCKY

When the Robert Wood Johnson Foundation chooses a setting for its Culture of Health conference, it wants to make sure participants learn something about the challenges and opportunities embedded in that place. Each location becomes a valuable case study, with conference sessions that highlight local pathways and challenges that are often unique yet also representative of other areas.

The first conference, held in Baltimore in 2016, helped pull back the curtain on urban life and the difficulties inherent in establishing a Culture of Health in a struggling but optimistic city. Louisville was a rich setting for the 2017 conference, given the health-impacting inequities and determined efforts to overcome them that exist at both the city and state levels.

This section captures the complexity of the 2017 conference host site. With highlights from two vigorous conference panels—one focused on the urban core of Louisville and one on the state's rural region of central Appalachia—it portrays stark health, economic, and political contrasts while calling out commonalities in urban and rural settings.

Louisville has a leg up over many other parts of the state because it has a number of major employers, including United Parcel Service, Humana Inc., and GE Appliances, as well as a healthy tourism industry fueled in part by the Louisville Slugger Museum and Factory and the Muhammad Ali Center.

Eastern Kentucky, by contrast, is starved for economic development. The consequences are dramatically illustrated in the *County Health Rankings & Roadmaps*, where measures of health factors (including health behavior, clinical care, social and economic factors, and the physical environment) and health outcomes show that the 30 counties ranked lowest in the state virtually all cluster on the eastern side.[1]

The state as a whole is considerably whiter than Louisville and has a much smaller black population. There are significant political differences as well. Louisville is in a sense a "blue dot within a red state," with a progressive mayor and a city council controlled by the Democrats. Kentucky is currently led by a Republican governor who is seeking a waiver of many provisions of Medicaid after its expansion had been approved by his predecessor, a Democrat.

Despite their geographic distance and demographic and political contrasts, many people in both urban and rural settings have limited opportunities, and access to all the elements of a healthy life is not spread equitably across the state. The average income of the top 1 percent of Kentucky residents is almost 17 times greater than the average for all residents.[2]

If inequity is a common denominator, the two regions share something more hopeful as well—the power of determined communities that believe they can move from problems and despair to possibilities and hope and who are putting their shoulders to the wheel to make that happen. The two chapters in this section look at how they are both trying to find their way toward a Culture of Health.

"The Louisville Story" describes the steps taken to build a healthy city from the perspective of public and private sector leaders. Mayor Greg Fischer sees compassion, lifelong learning, and health as the pillars of progress, and the city is supporting a package of programs in an effort to advance on all of those fronts. "A View from Appalachia" looks at the challenges of rural Kentucky from the ground up. Presenters describe the partnerships they have formed to counter the sense of hopelessness that has pervaded the landscape and what they are doing to drive toward new possibilities.

The Louisville Story

ERIK EAKER, MHA
Director, Population Health Initiatives, Humana Inc.

GREG FISCHER
Mayor, City of Louisville, Kentucky

BRANDY N. KELLY PRYOR, PHD, MA
Director, Center for Health Equity, Louisville Metro Government

TED SMITH, PHD
Chief Executive Officer, Revon Systems Inc.

A visitor who heads to one of the big hotels in downtown Louisville and enjoys the lively restaurants nearby might be forgiven for thinking this is a thriving modern city. And indeed some $4 billion in private development is planned by the summer of 2018, according to the Louisville Downtown Partnership. Historic districts are coming back to life block by block as apartments are rehabilitated, and Waterfront Park, once a wasteland of abandoned industrial buildings, now receives 2 million visitors a year.

But there remain inequities. Louisville's "Ninth Street Divide" still symbolically and geographically divides the city between east and west, black and white, rich and poor. A single data point from the Center for Health Equity could not be starker: the gap in life expectancy between residents of the lowest and highest income areas in Louisville can be as much as 16 to 18 years.[1]

Many years ago, Louisville leaders set out to explore how differences in place were fostering that kind of profound inequity. The city has since launched a slate of new initiatives with the shared goal of becoming one of the healthiest cities in the country by 2020, no matter where its citizens live. These ongoing efforts to acknowledge disparities and redefine health for its citizens were recognized when Louisville received the Robert Wood Johnson Foundation (RWJF) Culture of Health Prize in 2016.

A Journey Begins With Disparities

Like many major cities in the United States, Louisville has a long history of racial divides and segregated neighborhoods. But the profound inequities created by such divisions came into full view in 2003, when the city merged with surrounding Jefferson County, creating a metropolitan area that now has some 750,000 people. White residents made up about 74 percent of Louisville Metro's population, while black residents living in a cluster of neighborhoods in the western region represented about 20 percent of the population.

The merger in many ways accomplished its goals of increasing government efficiency and spurring economic development. According to panel moderator Ted Smith, who served as Louisville's first chief innovation officer from 2011 to 2016, the economy is now highly diversified. Along with a well-established food and beverage industry, Louisville is home to a major United Parcel Service hub, headquarters more aging-care companies than any other city in the country, and has an emerging business services industry.

But the merger also put an unexpected spotlight on one critical fact: the core urban communities lag significantly behind the suburbs in many measures of health and well-being. Today, the associated opportunities of economic development still benefit the more suburban areas of the city far more than they do places like west Louisville. The disparities in income, lifestyles, access to health care, and life expectancies within the new Louisville Metro area remain stark.

Brandy N. Kelly Pryor, director of the city's Center for Health Equity, highlighted this divide. Her data show that the gap in life expectancy between residents of the lowest and highest income areas in the city can be nearly 16 years. What's more, she noted, more than 63 percent of Louisville residents live in neighborhoods with a life expectancy below the national average of 79 years. Almost 32 percent of black residents are in fair or poor health, and one in four children live in poverty, as do one in seven adults.[2] According to 2014 data from the Network Center for Community Change, median incomes in some west Louisville neighborhoods are less than half the median for Jefferson County.[3]

Significant disparities in personal safety and educational opportunities exist in the city, too. In fact, one of the most sobering statistics in Louisville may be that its most dangerous neighborhoods have violent crime rates up to 35 times higher than the safest neighborhoods.[4]

Where life expectancy plummets, discrepancies in lifestyle and services are evident. In the poorest areas of the city, between 38 percent and 69 percent of households have no car, compared to 0 percent to 5.4 percent of households in the wealthiest suburbs. The same graph showed that residents in the poorest areas live without easy access to a major, full-service grocery store.

"We're talking about the social determinants of health when we're talking about transportation," Kelly Pryor explained. "We know that transportation correlates with income rates in the city. And where you see that people don't have cars, you will see that there is also a lack of grocery stores."

Asking New Questions About Health

Louisville's journey to create a Culture of Health began after the city-county merger, when city officials pledged to become a more compassionate, equitable city for all. The Greater Louisville Project was soon created to provide research and data that support civic actions to meet this goal and help redefine health as "what we are every day."

A Brookings Institution report, commissioned by the project, identified six "deep drivers of change" that would help the newly merged Louisville Metro region move forward: primary education, postsecondary education, economic development, quality neighborhoods, investments in working families, and balanced growth. The Greater Louisville Project soon honed in on education, jobs, and quality of place as three factors that make a city competitive and attractive to businesses and citizens. It would soon add a fourth: health.

> *Our goal as a community is to be the place where everyone can have the opportunity to meet their full potential and everyone has the opportunity to thrive.*
> *—Greater Louisville Project*

Since taking office in 2010 and winning reelection in 2014, Mayor Greg Fischer has leaned heavily on one unique aspect of Louisville's effort to rethink the city's health: the Center for Health Equity. The first such center in the country within a city health department, it is designed to challenge the way officials ask questions about health.

Established in 2006 as a division of the Metro Department of Public Health and Wellness, the Center for Health Equity asked whether investing in schools, improving housing, integrating neighborhoods, and providing better jobs could be "health strategies" with the same power as strategies to influence smoking, diet, and exercise. Concluding the answer was "yes," the center began to support projects, policies, and research to address the correlation between health, longevity, and socioeconomic status—with a particular focus on those who have been historically and institutionally marginalized.

> *We have a moral responsibility to impact public health goals. And to improve health without understanding social justice issues is not possible.*
> *—Brandy N. Kelly Pryor*

Kelly Pryor, who was named director of the center in 2015, used the analogy of a tree to describe the center's vision. She concluded that health outcomes and chronic conditions, such as diabetes and obesity, are in the tree's leaves, while social determinants, such as education, housing, and transportation, are in its roots. For instance, in addition to the disparities in car ownership, the city's mass transit bus services cater daily to 50,000 disproportionately lower income riders, according to Smith.

"So let's talk about why transportation is the way it is in certain parts of the city," said Kelly Pryor. "Let's talk about education and housing. And we're going even deeper, now, to talk about racism, sexism, homophobia, and other social determinants of equity, which are in the soil."

Conversations around racial and health inequities, she noted, require historical perspective. For instance, many of the structural and institutional barriers that still impact Louisville's deeply segregated housing areas are rooted in practices that happened decades ago. She referenced the Redlining Map project, launched by the city in February 2017 to address the practice of denying loans in certain neighborhoods because of race or socioeconomic characteristics. The project uses maps and data to show how redlining impacted Louisville in the past and how it still plays a role today.[5]

"We're talking about racism that might have happened in 1937, and how that's now impacting health in 2017," she said. "So that conversation around race and health started a long time before, but we're finally at a place politically as well as socially in our country where governments are starting to say, 'What can we do to challenge this conversation?'"

For the first time in the city's history, Kelly Pryor points out, both "health" and "equity" are included along with "education, jobs, and quality of place" as important benchmarks in comprehensive plans now being developed for Louisville's future.

She is making sure that the Center for Health Equity "is right at the forefront of all those conversations. When we talk about improving the health of all people, we can't do that without really tackling and understanding the social justice issues that are affecting our city. We are changing the way in which we ask questions about health. We are changing questions about what individuals are doing to impact health behavior, and challenging what the structures have done in some ways to inflict violence on individuals."

Three Values Help Define Solutions

Fischer was an admitted political outlier when he was elected mayor. "I'm a businessman and an entrepreneur with the heart of a social worker," he joked.

To guide his commitment to fostering a community in which everyone has the opportunity to thrive, he asked some unusual questions: "What makes a city tick? How do you make decisions? What's the filter that you run all decisions through?"

Since coming to office, Fischer has embraced three values as the pillars that support Louisville's Culture of Health agenda: compassion, lifelong learning, and health.

Creating a More Compassionate Community

On November 11, 2011, Louisville declared itself a Compassionate City and committed to a 10-year Compassionate City Campaign. Fischer and the city defined compassion as something that "impels us to work tirelessly to alleviate the suffering of our fellow creatures, to dethrone ourselves from the center of our world and put another there, and to honor the inviolable sanctity of every single human being, treating everybody, without exception, with absolute justice, equity and respect."

Fischer admitted that this concept of compassion "kind of freaked people out when I said it. Because they think, 'Well, that sounds kind of soft. You're supposed to be tough, you're supposed to be a politician.' And I said, 'well, my experience is it's harder for people to be compassionate than it is to be cynical or angry or a skeptic from the couch. So we need to exercise that compassion muscle.'"

> We must create a more compassionate city, where neighbor cares for neighbor, friend for friend, stranger for stranger. Our city defines compassion as providing citizens the tools and support necessary to reach their full human potential.
> —Mayor Greg Fischer

The city's compassionate campaign has resulted in a wide range of projects, including the "Give a Day" volunteer initiative, mentoring programs for adults and children alike, community beautification, and clean-up projects. Louisville's "Heart of Gold" monthly program recognizes compassion efforts that range from shoveling snow for an elderly neighbor to corporate sponsorship of Habitat for Humanity housing projects.

The city sees its compassion mission playing out in scenarios as diverse as the Louisville population itself. There's compassion when a group of young mothers gather with their children in a Louisville park to support one another's recovery from substance abuse. There's compassion when an evicted veteran quickly obtains a Section 8 low-income housing voucher in a city that has eliminated veteran homelessness. There's compassion when young professionals raise money to provide field trips for at-risk children and youth. And in Louisville's Compassionate Schools program, where educators strive to integrate social and emotional learning, wellness, nutrition, and mindfulness into the elementary school curriculum, there is compassion for how each student spent the previous night, with questions asked about their lives like, "Did they have enough to eat, feel loved by caregivers, sleep in safe surroundings?"

In February 2017, when the city launched efforts to address redlining, Fischer considered that an important "compassion play," too. "Most people—especially most white people—don't understand these structural and institutional barriers that have been in place." The redlining project and its interactive, online tools "is an easy way the government can just talk about facts and data so that people can understand history and maybe say, 'Okay, I understand that better now.' Or, if you're a lender you can say, 'We need to focus in a particular area' to make sure whatever product we might be selling is accessible to all and that we're putting an equitable playing field out there for everybody to succeed with."

The city's reputation for compassion prompted a 2013 visit from the Dalai Lama of Tibet, a spiritual leader committed to compassion, forgiveness, and tolerance, who has since developed a continuing relationship with the city. And, in 2016, the Charter of Compassion named Louisville a Model City for Compassion for the fifth year in a row, the largest city in America with that distinction.

Promoting Lifelong Learning

Lifelong learning is another core commitment in Louisville, said Fischer. "It's this notion that if we can live in a city where everybody is constantly learning, everybody has got a chance to succeed." Many of the city's lifelong learning initiatives are specifically designed to close the gap between advantaged and disadvantaged families.

For example, 55,000 Degrees, launched in 2010, aims to make sure at least half of the adults in Louisville have an associate, bachelor's, or higher degree by 2020 and that 85 percent of high school graduates are enrolled in postsecondary degree programs by 2020.

That goal is consistent with findings that people with higher degrees have higher incomes, are less likely to ever smoke or to be obese, have fewer divorces, and are more likely to exercise. Increasing the number of citizens with higher degrees will also address a shortage in Louisville's workforce.[6] The dozens of business, education, and community-based partners that support the program have already seen significant progress: the number of high school students who attended college grew from 45 percent in 2012 to 63 percent in 2016. "When we started we were below the national average by 10 percent," said Fischer. "Now we're above the national average."

Another initiative, Cradle to Career, launched in 2014, is designed to incorporate learning before students enter their first classroom and to continue it long after graduation. A key goal is to ensure that more than 75 percent of kindergarten students are prepared to enter school by 2020.

According to Fischer, a disadvantaged child—and that describes more than 50 percent of Louisville's first graders—will show up in kindergarten three years behind a child from an advantaged family. "Now, how do we expect those kids to catch up?" he asked. "Our society seems awfully content to pay for the cost of that later, through incarceration, through crime, whatever it might be. Our system is turned upside down." In the three years since the city's kindergarten readiness program was developed, with support from Metro United Way, Fischer said the number of children ready for kindergarten has jumped from 35 percent to 51 percent.

The Cradle to Career program also aims to have every student reading at grade level by the end of third grade and to achieve a 90 percent high school graduation rate. Training and programming are also provided to help residents succeed in the regional marketing, tech, and health care sectors.

Creating a Healthier City

The third value that Fischer ascribes to a city's Culture of Health is, naturally, health. "How can we be a healthier city?" Fischer asked. "Obviously, people think about physical health, and I'm glad to see more talk about mental health. The other aspect of health is environmental health. How do we make sure our air, our water, our soil are improving? How can we be loud and proud about that?"

Fischer highlighted three efforts to create a healthier, more equitable Louisville:

- **Healthy Louisville.** Funded by Louisville Metro Public Health and Wellness, the Healthy Louisville 2020 Plan "makes sure we are looking at equity in all ways, and looking at that through a policy lens."
- **AIR Louisville.** With more than 2,000 "citizen scientists" using asthma inhalers with a tracking device, the AIR Louisville project is capturing data both to help individuals manage their own asthma and to gather aggregated information to improve public health. The problem is widespread. Nationally, about 8 percent of the population suffers with asthma; in Louisville that rate is closer to 13 percent.[7]

    When the sensor-laden inhalers pinpoint places where a preponderance of asthma attacks occur, the city can mitigate the problem with "vegetative medicine"—that is, trees and shrubs. Research has linked an abundance of trees, and the improvements they generate in air quality, to lower asthma rates.

The data also help to identify citizen scientists who are using their inhalers dramatically more than other users; the program then partners this subgroup with a respiratory therapist. When that one-to-one connection is made, these individuals have seen an 80 percent reduction in the use of inhalers.

- **Pivot to Peace and other initiatives that address violence.** The city of Louisville now looks at violence through a public health lens, said Fischer. "Violence is a learned behavior. Violence can be looked at as a contagion that spreads through a community. How do you isolate that contagion and eliminate what is obviously a severe health crisis?"

One program, Pivot to Peace, works with people who have been hospitalized with a gunshot wound or a stabbing injury. Counselors work to show these victims of violence that there is a "different path forward if they will put down weapons and find a way to be productive citizens," Fischer explained.

Other programs foster collaboration. Weekly neighborhood Peace Walks with residents and police help both sides share ideas on how to make the city safer. Project H.E.A.L. (Health. Equity. Art. Learning.), a five-year effort that uses the arts to help residents look for solutions, incorporates drum circles in the Smoketown neighborhood of Louisville, an area of the city with high poverty and crime rates. A photovoice exhibit, featuring the photographs and written observations of west Louisville residents, leads to community meetings to help pinpoint ways to reduce violence in this neighborhood, which has one of the highest violent crime rates in the city.

> *There is going to be tragedy in all of our cities. The question is, "How do we respond when these adverse events take place?" Do we turn on each other, or do we come together as a community? And I'm happy to say that we come together as a community.*
> *—Mayor Greg Fischer*

A Healthier City Measured by Healthy Days

Another initiative that seeks to better understand the community's well-being while relying on data is Louisville's Bold Goal initiative. A collaborative effort with Humana Inc., the health insurance company headquartered in Louisville, the initiative aims to ensure that Louisville is 20 percent healthier by 2020, as measured by a tool called Healthy Days. This is a health-related quality-of-life measure developed and validated by the Centers for Disease Control and Prevention.[8]

The Bold Goal initiative, already launched or planned for 10 cities around the country, started in Louisville in 2015. Data comes from multiple sources—insurance claims, social determinants of health frameworks, in-depth interviews, focus groups with community members, and a clinical town hall, where organizations committed to addressing health challenges can collaborate.

The initiative tracks not only physical and mental health but utilization rates, health care costs, appropriate use of medicine, and health care markers associated with diabetes, congestive heart failure, coronary artery disease, behavioral health, and upper respiratory health. It also recognizes that social isolation, loneliness, and food insecurity are important social determinants of health. By 2020, the initiative aims to move from a baseline of 9.0 unhealthy days to 7.2—an increase of 1.8 "healthy" days for every individual.

> *We discovered that Healthy Days was not only important as a measure of physical and mental health, but it was also highly correlated to health care utilization, medication adherence, and health care costs, things we could prove with our claims data.*
> —*Erik Eaker*

Reflections on Opportunities and Solutions

In closing remarks, Fischer circled back to emphasize the value of incorporating compassion into city development and operations. He emphasized that cities are responsible for much of the growth and innovation that contributes to the country's gross domestic product (GDP) and can play a key role in convening cross-sector groups from health, arts, business, and the community. "There is value in viewing one another as partners," he said.

Smith returned again to data, asking Kelly Pryor, "Where has data made a big difference? Where have you been able to get a conversation moving and get people fired up?" Kelly Pryor immediately offered several examples of initiatives that use data to "tell a more dynamic story, to get to granular-level data that we might not be able to see in our Census tracts."

A robust story may emerge, for example, by layering the locations of grocery stores and transportation over patterns of life expectancy and racial segregation. Using these "story maps" also encourages community conversation, allowing quantitative data to become qualitative. The ability to turn data into storytelling has also inspired partnerships with organizations such as IDEAS xLab, which focuses on the arts, and the Youth Violence Prevention Research Center, which helps tell stories of young people.

Audience member Andrea Levere, president of Prosperity Now, an organization that promotes financial security as a way to move people out of poverty, asked Kelly Pryor if her work addresses financial insecurity. Kelly Pryor noted that it does, pointing out that data show those who are most affected by violence tend to be those who are most financially insecure. The so-called Golden Ticket initiative in Louisville helps fast-track victims of violence into job opportunities with local corporations and nonprofit organizations through the city's KentuckianaWorks program.

Too, Kelly Pryor pointed to a recent report by the Greater Louisville Project that embraced the Brookings Institution's framework of financial insecurity as more than just income. "It is wealth, it's education, it's housing, it's how many people live in your neighborhood who are also financially insecure. We're trying to tackle all of these determinants to create a better, more secure financial community in Louisville."

Camara Jones, MD, PhD, MPH, a senior fellow at Morehouse School of Medicine and the past president of the American Public Health Association, pointed out that Louisville had operationalized two of what she considered the three key principles for achieving health equity: (1) valuing all individuals and populations equally (accomplished through the city's work on compassion) and (2) recognizing and rectifying historical injustices (accomplished through the city's work to rectify redlining and other historical injustices). But she asked whether Louisville had achieved the third principle of health equity—providing resources according to need.

Not yet, admitted Kelly Pryor, adding that the city's efforts to get there are "intentional." Under the direction of the chief equity officer, the city is developing a racial equity toolkit with a five-city cohort called Racial Equity Here through a partnership between the Government Alliance on Race and Equity and Living Cities Foundation, designed to help determine who is most financially burdened by social policies and to serve as a guide to reallocating resources. She also gave a shout-out to the city's new Fair Housing Assessment being developed by Louisville's Human Resource Commission, which will look at housing and allocate resources to those who need it most.

One of the challenges, Kelly Pryor admitted, is that "there is a mindset that equity is a zero-sum game, as in there are not going to be enough pieces of the pie for all of us." Instead of the pie imagery, she embraces the concept of universal design, where amenities like curb cuts have shared value that benefits everyone, not just people with disabilities. "That is the language that we want to bring to resource allocation in Louisville—that we're raising the bar for everyone and creating a Louisville Metro where we all thrive."

A View from Appalachia

GABRIELA ALCALDE, MPH, DRPH
Managing Director for Equity and Health, Richmond Memorial Health Foundation

JARED ARNETT, MBA
Founding Executive Director, Shaping Our Appalachian Region, Inc.

ADRIENNE BUSH
Executive Director, Hazard Perry County Community Ministries

GILBERT LIU, MD
Medical Director, Kentucky Department of Medicaid Services

> *I hear people talk about white privilege a lot on the East Coast. . . . It made me start thinking that maybe in eastern Kentucky, we're not white.*
> —*Resident of rural Kentucky*

Some 200 miles from Louisville lies the rural landscape of Appalachia in eastern Kentucky, where poverty rates are among the highest in the country. Six counties in coal country rank among the bottom 10 counties nationwide, based on measures of education, household income, unemployment, disabilities, life expectancy, and obesity.[1] In these same six counties, between 25 and 31 percent of the population are ranked as being in "fair or poor" health, according to *County Health Rankings & Roadmaps* data.[2]

Vast tracts of land in this hard-hit region are inhabited by people isolated from education and training, job opportunities, health care, and social services. Stories and statistics from this predominantly white region belie the myth that poverty is largely the provenance of populations of color in urban areas. They also highlight the unmistakable influence of class as a determining feature of how well people do.

But despite its very real deficits, rural Kentucky remains rich in culture, tradition, and family connection, and it is a "treasure trove of lore, stories, and wisdom," said Gilbert Liu. To guide a conversation about the landscape, the

people, and the forward-looking initiatives under way in the region, Liu introduced three "inspired leaders who offer pearls of insights that should be enacted
into broad-ranging improvements in health policy."

Taking Ownership in Appalachia

Jared Arnett, who calls himself "a boy from the head of a holler," leads Shaping
Our Appalachian Region (SOAR), which views itself as "a holistic champion for
a 21st-century Appalachia." Founded in 2015 as a bipartisan effort by Kentucky's
Democratic governor and a Republican congressman from the area, SOAR seeks
to "revitalize and reimagine and champion new ideas around rebuilding an economic base in eastern Kentucky."

For 50 years, task forces, blue ribbon panels, and commissions have analyzed
the region, yet its vast needs have only intensified. Between 2006 and 2016, total
employment across 22 counties fell by almost 45,000 jobs. Floyd County, one
of Kentucky's least prosperous, has 28 jobs for every 100 adults while the relatively more affluent Fayette County, where the state capitol of Lexington sits,
offers 60 jobs to 100 adults. Unless tens of thousands of new jobs are added to
the rolls, it will be almost impossible to move the needle on economic progress
in a significant way.

The SOAR Attitude

SOAR was created as a venue for the region's institutions, businesses, leaders, and
citizens to collaborate and innovate. Following an unexpectedly well-attended
summit meeting in December 2013, 10 working groups were formed to hold
listening sessions across eastern Kentucky, and the framework for a partnership
organization began to be erected. The needs were enormous, and funding was
sparse. "We were essentially given zero authority and zero money to spend and
an expectation to fix 60 years' worth of problems in six months," said Arnett,
somewhat tongue-in-cheek.

After assessing the work already under way in eastern Kentucky, the SOAR
team identified deep fragmentation and poor communication as core problems.
Some exciting work was happening, but nobody knew what anyone else was
doing, and everybody had separate strategies. "It was just a disorganized, chaotic
mess," Arnett recalls. "It became clear that the region did not necessarily need
one more program in health care or workforce development or entrepreneurship, but rather an overarching vision to guide action."

SOAR began crafting such a vision, assembling a diverse set of players to
move it forward. Arnett recalls attending a board meeting where the governor,

a congressman, and a chief executive officer of the community college system joined banking and hospital executives, grassroots representatives, and even members of a high school team that had won national recognition for a computer app. "You've got all these people coming together with one mind, and it has become pretty powerful," he said.

Increasingly, they are able to move together on many fronts, believing that while "there is not a silver bullet" to fix eastern Kentucky, "there are a lot of silver BBs." SOAR's Regional Blueprint for Economic Growth, released in November 2016, connects its existing programs to three strategies: "drive action, be the champion, and grow the team." Seven goals build on that structure:

1. Increase the availability of affordable high-speed broadband through fiber to businesses and residents, and increase adoption rates throughout the SOAR region.
2. Develop a regional workforce to be competitive in the digital economy and other emerging industries.
3. Create more small businesses and expand existing ones within the region by taking full advantage of the digital economy.
4. Reduce the physical and economic impact of obesity, diabetes, and substance abuse.
5. Increase the amount of industrial employment, which includes manufacturing, natural resources, processing, and distribution, by expanding existing companies and attracting new ones.
6. Create a local foods movement by connecting local producers to markets for their products both within and outside the region.
7. Establish Kentucky's Appalachian region as a tourism destination.

These goals are interconnected, reflecting SOAR's commitment to breaking down silos. For example, a telehealth initiative crosses the boundaries of health care, broadband technology, and economic development by offering residents critical access to medical specialists as well as training at a local technical college that can lead to a Telehealth Technician Certificate.

Scaling Up

It is not just about creating jobs, it's about creating a system that can continually do that and be sustainable.

—Jared Arnett

Ultimately, SOAR is as much an attitude as it is an initiative. In communities that have felt hopeless, partners are inspiring people to dream bigger and helping them realize they are not alone. SOAR spreads the impact of its four-person staff through strategic efforts intended to be both transformational and scalable. "We want to provide a model that then people can take and run with," Arnett said. "We want to support thousands of people doing that in the region, and elevate the awareness of what they are doing."

Arnett is convinced that the future of Appalachian Kentucky hinges on its ability to embrace technology and join the twenty-first-century digital economy. "Access to broadband absolutely changes every sector, every opportunity," he said, recalling the eye-opening moment when Amazon officials told him that the digital economy offered 18 million jobs. The possibility that local people could remain in their own communities and be trained for some of that work has become infused in much of SOAR's plans.

One of SOAR's signature activities is an annual Innovation Summit. Based on online applications, 141 people were selected to showcase solutions to local problems at the third summit, held in 2016 (40 projects were health-related). The governor spent the entire day at the event, which drew 1,200 people.

In the same spirit, the Massachusetts Institute of Technology (MIT) facilitated the MIT Appalachian Health Hack-a-Thon in October 2016, where 19 teams presented novel ideas—such as an app that alerts responders to a suspected overdose and another that draws attention to the need for prediabetic screening among Medicaid patients.

TechHire Eastern Kentucky (TEKY) is another burgeoning collaboration, and has transformed the narrative around the type of worker that can succeed in today's digital economy. Fifty-five trainees, culled from 850 applicants, were selected for an intensive paid internship designed to train them as coders. Thirty-five completed the programs, earned certificates, and are now employed. Their comments on social media sing with enthusiasm: "Proud to be part of this adventure into the future." "Thank you so much to all involved for believing in us!!!"

> *This is truly the beginning of something great and wonderful.*
> —TEKY trainee

With a $3.5 million grant from the Appalachian Regional Commission, TEKY 2 is now ready to launch. The program will be expanded to three more community colleges, with private sector partners, including Amazon, coming in to conduct the training.

An online network, structured much like LinkedIn and Facebook, but targeted specifically at Kentucky's rural communities, is now live, helping to foster the connections and collaborative initiatives that are foundational to SOAR's work. But instilling a sense of ownership is not an easy job. Arnett recalls one post on social media that hinted at lingering passivity: "Is this simply going to be another feel good political thing or is it going to help families? We stand back and watch."

That last line represents the kind of thinking "that we're trying to push against in eastern Kentucky," Arnett explained. "The question I ask at every presentation is, 'Will we own it or are we going to be another organization that's waiting for Frankfort [Kentucky] or DC to figure it out and fix it? Are we going to figure out how to do it on our own?"

Arnett returns again and again to his conviction that broadband access can foster tremendous opportunities for the region. "Technology can disrupt the cab industry and the hotel industry. We think it can also disrupt rural poverty," he declares. "We think it can disrupt the economic challenges within this region, so we're trying to integrate it across the board."

The Unique Challenges of Rural Housing

We can implement housing-first policies that get people into housing. Their outcomes, particularly around health, are going to be much, much better if they are in stable housing, rather than in an emergency shelter.
—Adrienne Bush

Just as technology is the focal point for SOAR, housing is Adrienne Bush's overarching concern, because she views it as the foundation for individual and community health. "Housing is one of the things that we take for granted, but if you don't have it, it's really hard to achieve anything else," she said. Bush heads the Homeless and Housing Coalition of Kentucky, a statewide coalition that addresses affordable housing and the housing needs of special populations.

Housing touches all four action areas within the Culture of Health Action Framework, she explained:

- **Making health a shared value:** Good housing stock is an essential characteristic of a healthy community, but the supply across rural America is inadequate. Much of it is aging, a high percentage is outdated manufactured homes, and some is tied up in various legal disputes. The focus of development investments and public subsidies to bolster housing options should be determined with local input, said Bush. For example, many initiatives are designed to promote home ownership, but adequate rental housing is the greater priority in some settings. "The opportunity here is creating a sense of community and investing in different types of housing, based on a community's needs and wants," she explained.

- **Fostering cross-sector collaboration:** In recent years, public policies have encouraged service providers to take a broader view of the continuum of supports necessary to house people and especially to keep them housed. The federal Department of Housing and Urban Development (HUD) is also paying more attention to local control, asking communities, "What do you need in order to get people housed quickly and make sure that homelessness is brief, rare, and nonrecurring?"

  The recognition that homeless populations require wraparound services from many types of providers, coupled with the resource limitations that characterize rural Kentucky, has fostered partnerships out of sheer necessity. For example, the Kentucky Interagency Council on Homelessness engages agencies involved with veterans' affairs, criminal justice, education and workforce development, behavioral health, and more.

  But siloes remain, and it is still too easy for organizations without a health mission to set a concern for health aside. Kentucky is also challenged by its sparse population, spread across a wide geographic area, and the jurisdictional issues that complicate governance and decision-making in the state's 120 counties.

- **Creating healthier, more equitable communities:** The package of challenges that need to be addressed to drive toward greater equity include addressing youth and family homelessness and meeting the special needs of aging populations and the nontraditional, nonnuclear families that are increasingly common. Another priority is to affirmatively further HUD's fair housing requirements. In addition to meeting other civil rights provisions, HUD-funded projects are explicitly barred from putting up "any barriers based on marital status, gender, or gender identity."

  Supporting the home ownership development activities of nonprofit organizations in the area and protecting renters' rights are other pathways toward more equitable communities. For example, the Homeless and Housing Coalition of Kentucky advocates for state adoption of the Uniform Residential Landlord Tenant Act, which spells out a landlord's obligations to ensure basic habitability of rental units.

- **Strengthening integration of health services and systems:** Access to care is a necessary precondition for effectively integrating services and systems. That means having an adequate number of providers; preserving health insurance options, such as the Medicaid expansion under the Affordable Care Act; and ensuring the availability of transportation so that people can actually reach the care they need.

  Using a common assessment tool and coordinating entry into housing services across systems are essential integration strategies for the homeless population. Traditionally, an individual has had to be designated "street homeless" to be granted a slot in an emergency shelter. From there, Bush explained, "If you were good and you were really compliant with the program, we might let you into our transitional shelter. And then after that, we might talk about providing a rental voucher."

That approach has changed, based on the work of Dennis Culhane at the University of Pennsylvania and others, which supports the foundational value of "housing first" policies.[3] Increasingly, services are also being prioritized on the basis of vulnerability rather than on a "first-come, first-served" basis.

Driving Toward Equity

What does it take to build rural health and equity? Drawing from the Culture of Health Action Framework, as Bush did in the housing context, Gabriela Alcalde explored the many angles to that question more broadly. She opened her presentation by describing the Foundation for Healthy Kentucky, which is both a grantmaking and an operating foundation that works on the policy level to address the unmet health care needs of Kentuckians. Improving access to care, reducing health risks and disparities, and promoting health equity are particular areas of focus.

Because people approach these concepts with different assumptions, Alcalde offered her own definitions, distinguishing *disparities*, a term that recognizes the existence of difference but does not place value on it, from *inequities*, which are "unfair, unnecessary, and avoidable." Three key principles help sharpen her perspective:

- Inequities are disparities that are preventable and unfair.
- Decreasing disparities is part of working toward health equity, but it is not enough.
- Equity requires understanding and addressing the root causes that lead to disparities.

Although most efforts to promote greater equity recognize the special needs of populations that have experienced socioeconomic disadvantages or historical injustice, the realities of rural communities are too often overlooked. The neglect of Appalachia, where the economy has historically been dominated by mining and other resource extraction techniques, has been particularly acute. "There have been historical

Equity is about fairness, it is not about differences.
—Gabriela Alcalde

exploitation and experiences that we don't traditionally identify with white populations in the U.S.," Alcalde said.

How Shared Values Shape Policies

Our values shape our policies, and in turn our policies influence and shape our values.

—Gabriela Alcalde

Although sound policy rests partly on a foundation of strong data, Alcalde urged that adequate attention also be directed to qualitative influences and lived experience. "The failure to include the community from the beginning is often the downfall of very well-though- out and generously funded projects," she said. "That has to be a mistake we do not continue to make."

Listening to the community means engaging not only local leaders but ordinary local people as well. "Often times, what we'll find is they really do understand why things are happening and they understand how to change them."

To build on shared values, the influence of social determinants and economic inequality on health needs to be explicitly acknowledged. Clinicians, front-office staff at provider facilities, and others need to be educated about how health connects with housing, transportation, education, and the built environment and consider "how our entire environment receives, or does not receive, our community." Alcalde calls for metrics that look broadly at return on investment over time, rather than expecting prevention to immediately cut costs. "Equity is good for everyone," she said. "It is good for the health of the community and it is good for the health of the economy, and that's a long-term investment. We should not be looking at immediate monetary dollar values to be returned on prevention investments."

The Power of Cross-Sector Collaborations

Recognizing that "health happens everywhere," policies and assumptions need to be in place that allow, encourage, and sustain cross-sector collaborations. Alcalde identified some of the necessary elements:

- **Supporting staff to participate in the sometimes-uncomfortable process of building relationships and trust.** "They need to be encouraged, to know that this is an expectation and part of their job," said Alcalde.
- **Flexible funding.** A broad view of the interrelated influences on health allows for investments that cross sectors (for example, using housing funds to pay for transportation systems that can sustain people in their homes).

- **Systems built to communicate with one another.** Today's electronic health records make it very difficult to share information broadly, fostering silos instead of breaking them down.
- **Data sharing.** Within and outside government, de-identified data need to be bridged across sectors, so that economic, housing, education, health, and other indicators and outcomes can be analyzed. "We should be able to look at all that data together to get a complete picture and really have a comprehensive, holistic intervention," said Alcalde.
- **Allocating time, resources, and technical assistance to build local capacity** that can sustain community-driven coalitions beyond their current funding.

Building Healthier, More Equitable Communities

You need to look around the room, see who's missing and ask, "Why are they missing?" And we need to correct that.
—*Gabriela Alcalde*

Despite a hefty evidence base to guide strategies for building equitable communities, people often question the relevance of research findings from other settings. Alcalde bemoaned the common litany: "Well, that wasn't in Kentucky. Kentucky is different." While every community is indeed unique, there are opportunities to draw on available evidence in a modular fashion and custom-tailor it for local use. "There is no need to reinvent the wheel," she said.

The importance of involving the community from the outset is a paramount priority, one Alcalde would like to "bold-face and underline a thousand times. . . . We don't get to decide who the community is. We don't get to select who those representatives are, so it takes time." Among other overlooked populations, young people are often left out of youth- and child-centered work, with adult proxies consulted instead. Her strongly held view is that youth should be given opportunities to contribute in culturally competent, developmentally appropriate ways.

Alcalde bluntly stated that equity work cannot move forward without "speaking of the elephant in the room—and calling racism by its name." Euphemisms like "racial tensions" won't do the trick. "This country has severe problems with race and class, and we need to call them what they are."

Integrating Systems

Strengthening the rural infrastructure requires that systems and services become more integrated, both horizontally and vertically. Opportunities for greater streamlining, consistency, and integration exist in multiple realms: at various levels of government; among clinical care, public health, and social services; in the private and public sectors; and across policies and funding streams.

For example, a "no-wrong-door approach" recognizes that behavioral, physical, and oral health care need to be well-coordinated and responsive in order to serve individuals and families who lack the time or resources to wander a fragmented system. "If you show up at the first door and they tell you, 'Sorry, that's not here, that's down the street,' or 'No, they're not open,' you've just lost your opportunity to interact, to intercept, and to provide the necessary services and information," Alcalde warns. Although Medicaid managed care has somewhat improved Kentucky's ability to provide services seamlessly, regulatory barriers remain.

A team-based, interdisciplinary approach to care is particularly important in disadvantaged rural areas, but the task of integrating social and health services is complicated by administrative, programmatic, and financing silos. "We need to use our influence at the policy level to change funding streams so they are more flexible and we can be more creative," Alcalde emphasized. "There are definite human and economic costs to providing care in a fragmented way."

Beyond the fundamentals, such as ensuring access to insurance coverage and providers, breaking down barriers to care also means offering flexible service schedules, adequate transportation, opportunities to bring the children along, and workplace norms that encourage employers to provide time off. Cultural competence is another priority, one that is often overlooked when the native language of the populations involved is English. "One size does not fit all," said Alcalde, reminding her audience of the cultural uniqueness and diversity among Kentuckians and other rural people across the nation.

Engaging the business community is another component of integration and must be handled with delicacy. "You have to think very strategically about how you integrate that so you don't lose sight of your mission and what the common goal should be," Alcalde advises.

Collaborations often force participants to question their values and can cause unease—as they should. "Any time you diversify, there are going to be challenges and you have to create space for those challenges. If you invite people in, but you don't create the right atmosphere for them to be there, they are not going to stay."

All of these measures proceed best with a broad commitment to "health in all policies." That mindset creates the fertile ground in which integrated systems designed to improve access, decrease stigma, and remove barriers can emerge.

In wrapping up her talk, Alcalde returned to her definition of terms. "Equity is about fairness, and fairness is a moving target. It is not the same thing in every community, it is not the same thing over time. And what is fair from a population perspective may not feel fair to everyone." All of that creates discomfort and challenges, she acknowledges, but it also clarifies the way forward.

Reflections on the Rural Landscape

As he invited comments from the audience, moderator Liu underscored the passion that residents of rural Kentucky often have for their homeland. Many, he suggested, would readily turn down offers to move to urban areas like New York City or San Francisco, even knowing the move would likely lead to higher income and a longer life. "Things like family, faith, and grit are invaluable," he said. "They are impossible to monetize, but they are assets that need to be honored and revered and perpetuated."

Trené Hawkins, a program associate at RWJF, noted that recent discussions about rural people have tended to assume they are all poor and white, failing to recognize the communities of color, LGBTQ communities, aging populations, and many other marginalized people who also inhabit Appalachia. For that reason alone, Alcalde emphasized the need to look for leaders who understand their communities from the ground up. Taking a slightly different angle, Bush also stressed the value of seeking commonalities among populations, rather than focusing largely on differences.

Jessica Leifer, vice president of ideas42, which builds and tests interventions in partnership with community organizations, asked about the challenges of substance abuse, which is tearing apart so many families in the region. Acknowledging the widespread problem, Arnett returned the focus to the need for economic opportunities; without jobs, the prognosis for users after they complete treatment is bleak. The Addiction Recovery Center, one of SOAR's partners, offers a model of interest, training people in treatment to become peer counselors, which is a Medicaid-reimbursable service. The program guarantees participants jobs if they remain clean for a year.

Among other policy and clinical recommendations to meet rural needs in the face of the drug epidemic:

- Reinstate "kinship care" stipends to caregivers willing to step in when their relatives cannot tend to their children. Kentucky has put a moratorium on such stipends, which average about $300 a month, despite evidence that kinship care leads to better outcomes compared to foster care.
- Integrate behavioral and physical health services, and ensure that clinical care adheres to evidence-based guidelines. Liu called for a behavioral health

dictionary of services, accompanied by reimbursement codes, to reduce the huge variations in the nature and quality of available care.

- Use telemedicine, including remotely delivered counseling, to stretch inadequate provider networks.
- Design family-based approaches, such as treatment for both infants and the mothers who used substances during their pregnancies. Current systems tend to focus exclusively on individual treatment.

An audience member asked panelists for their perspectives on *Hillbilly Elegy,* the memoir by J. D. Vance that garnered so much public attention, especially after the 2016 presidential election. Several speakers questioned the way his personal story, with its tales of domestic violence and dysfunctional lifestyles, has come to be seen as a stand-in for all of Appalachia. "People don't realize there are a lot of different dynamics going on there," said Bush. "It's really hard for me to accept this as the entirety of the reality in eastern Kentucky."

Arnett acknowledged the reality of the memoir's storyline, but maintained his positive outlook. "Part of what we're trying to do is shift an entire culture. That's going to take a generation. How do we capture the generation going into middle school right now and start to shift the mindset?"

Gabriela Alcalde called Vance's book "a very narrow view, not a sociological or ethnographic perspective," and argued that positioning it as representative of an entire region "is profoundly harmful to eastern Kentucky and all of Appalachia. . . We would not do that for an immigrant population. If they did that for Latin-American immigrants, I would be hugely offended."

Those comments circled back to one of the session themes—that those whose voices are heard exert considerable influence on how policy unfolds and resources are allocated. For that reason, Alcalde urged funders and others in positions of influence to "question how they elevate single, biased views of entire regions or populations."

Epilogue

Continuing on the Journey Toward a Culture of Health

ABBEY K. COFSKY, MPH

Managing Director, Program, Robert Wood Johnson Foundation

MEGAN COLLADO, MPH

Director, Academy Health

PRIYA GANDHI, MS

Research Associate, Research-Evaluation-Learning,
Robert Wood Johnson Foundation

AMY GILLMAN, MPPM

Senior Program Officer, Program, Robert Wood Johnson Foundation

HEATHER HUGHES, MBA

Deputy Director and Vice President, Operations, YMCA of the USA

MICHELLE A. LARKIN, JD, MS, RN

Associate Chief of Staff, Robert Wood Johnson Foundation

JONATHAN LEVER, JD, MED

Executive Vice President and Chief Membership and Programs Officer, YMCA of the USA

KATIE E. WEHR, MPH

Senior Program Officer, Program, Robert Wood Johnson Foundation

The voices of researchers, practitioners, policymakers, and thought leaders captured in this volume have helped to tell the story of the Robert Wood Johnson Foundation's (RWJF) vision for a national Culture of Health. Launched in 2014, this vision lists health and well-being as priorities that are advanced by collaborators from all sectors, with a goal of enabling everyone to have a fair and just opportunity to live their healthiest and longest lives possible.

At Spotlight Health, the opening event of the Aspen Ideas Festival in June 2017, RWJF president and chief executive officer, Richard Besser, MD, described a Culture of Health as "making sure that all of those components are there to allow everyone to reach their full potential in terms of health and well-being." He stressed the importance of "pulling together parts of the community that haven't necessarily thought of their role as part of health, and get them to be part of the solutions."[1]

To support the realization of this vision, RWJF released the Culture of Health Action Framework in 2015. It identifies four interconnected Action Areas that incorporate the underlying principles of a Culture of Health and are intended to focus a multiplicity of initiatives and catalyze action by diverse individuals, communities, and organizations:

- **Making Health a Shared Value:** This Action Area puts the nation's goals about better health front and center; when individuals make health a priority in their actions and in policies and practices, national health and well-being will flourish.
- **Fostering Cross-Sector Collaboration to Improve Well-Being:** This Action Area highlights the importance of collaborations that include non-traditional collaborators to health and health care, such as business, law enforcement, transportation, education, and housing.
- **Creating Healthier, More Equitable Communities:** Not all places give people a fair opportunity for health and well-being. The goal of this Action Area is to improve the communities where people live, learn, work, and play so everyone has a fair chance to thrive.
- **Strengthening Integration of Health Services and Systems:** This Action Area encourages better balance and integration between medical treatment, public health, and social services, and demonstrates that high quality, efficient, and affordable care is critical to health and well-being.

Each Action Area includes a set of Drivers that help focus on progress at both national and community levels, along with a series of national, evidence-based Measures. The Action Framework is dynamic; while the Drivers will remain the same, the Measures will evolve. *Moving Forward Together*, a report published by RWJF, details the 2018 update to the Measures.[2]

In his Foreword to this book, Besser emphasized achieving health equity as critical to a Culture of Health. Underlying and vital to all components of the

Action Framework is the recognition that the vast inequities in opportunities for health and well-being for individuals across the nation must be addressed.

In the years since it launched the Culture of Health vision, RWJF has organized its programmatic work around four thematic areas, with Communications and Research-Evaluation-Learning serving important crosscutting functions:

- *Healthy Children, Healthy Weight* supports programs to address unacceptable disparities in an effort to ensure that all children attain good health.
- *Healthy Communities* looks to eliminate barriers to healthy choices and build healthier, more equitable communities.
- *Leadership for Better Health* develops and oversees many change leadership programs and works with the business sector.
- *Transforming Health and Health Care Systems* leads efforts to better coordinate and integrate health services and systems.

This epilogue offers a few examples of RWJF's initiatives that help advance health, well-being, and equity and a look at what RWJF is learning about early progress in building a Culture of Health.

Select Initiatives

This section offers three examples of RWJF's initiatives that plug into different points along the continuum of knowledge generation to action: building evidence through rigorous research, investing in initiatives that support communities, and working differently with long-term partners.

Building a Robust Evidence Base

Timely and objective research often relies on researchers' access to relevant data. But even when a dataset appropriate to help generate insights for a particular research question exists, it may be difficult for researchers to obtain. Proprietary datasets may be costly, and even open-access datasets may have technical and systems requirements that limit researchers' abilities to obtain and actually use them.

To reduce barriers to accessing longitudinal and large-scale datasets, RWJF developed the *Health Data for Action* (*HD4A*) program, which is supported by AcademyHealth. *HD4A* connects those holding the data to interested researchers, and looks to fund research studies that will use this data to glean actionable insights that can help answer research questions important to building a Culture of Health and inform health and related policies.

In 2017, *HD4A* provided successful applicants access to data from either athenahealth or the Health Care Cost Institute:

- **athenahealth** is a health care technology and services company connecting more than 85,000 medical providers from organizations of all sizes in both urban and rural communities across the nation. athenahealth providers are mostly based in outpatient care settings and include primary care providers, pediatricians, OB/GYNs, and other outpatient specialists.

  Under *HD4A*, athenahealth shared with researchers a de-identified dataset that included BMI readings from 2012 through 2016 for each visit to an athenahealth provider that was entered on its ambulatory electronic health record software at the point of care.
  - Study Spotlight: Evidence suggests that the food environment is associated with obesity risk, which is disproportionately present among racial minority populations. *HD4A* grantee Sara Bleich, PhD, Harvard College, is using athenahealth data to create a county-level measure of the restaurant environment to test whether changes in the restaurant environment lead to changes in obesity and whether this relationship varies by race/ ethnicity.
- **Health Care Cost Institute's** multiyear data included the annual health care claims for nearly 50 million people insured in the individual, group, or Medicare Advantage markets for 2008 through 2015.

  These data, contributed by three large national insurers—Aetna, Humana, and UnitedHealthcare—consisted of fully resolved, paid, de-identified medical and pharmacy claims.
  - Study Spotlight: Nearly half a million adolescents report nonmedical use of prescription opioids, and adolescents and young adults represent one of the most rapidly growing opiate abuse demographics. *HD4A* grantee Jason Hockenberry, PhD, Emory University, is using Health Care Cost Institute data to examine variation in pediatric prescribing practices nationwide and to assess the prevalence of new, persistent opioid acquisition in the pediatric population.

HD4A will continue to make large-scale, longitudinal datasets available to interested researchers from diverse sectors through different calls for proposals. Over time, the availability of large, vetted datasets will enable researchers to investigate novel ideas and consider visionary, blue-sky questions that otherwise may be unfeasible to study. Research, like that funded through *HD4A*, will open up avenues to innovation and help support RWJF's efforts to build a rigorous, transdisciplinary evidence base for a Culture of Health.

Investing to Build Healthy Communities

Mid-sized American cities face some of the nation's deepest challenges, with entrenched poverty, poor health, and a lack of investment. They also offer fertile ground for innovative cross-sector strategies that can improve health and boost local economies.

In May 2016, RWJF and Reinvestment Fund (a federally certified community development financial institution experienced in capital financing in low-income neighborhoods) announced the launch of *Invest Health*. The project brings together teams of diverse leaders from 50 mid-sized cities across the United States to catalyze and implement new strategies for increasing and leveraging private and public investments to accelerate improvements in neighborhoods facing the greatest barriers to better health.

Invest Health provides an opportunity to transform the way these local leaders work together to create solution-driven and diverse partnerships. The program is designed as an 18-month learning community intended to help city teams:

- Bring together disparate sectors to align around a vision for better health.
- Build lasting relationships that extend beyond the length of the program.
- Use data as a driver for change.
- Test potential solutions about how to best invest to achieve health equity.
- Advance systems-focused strategies specific to the built environment.
- Attract capital and unlock new sources of investment to improve health outcomes in low-income neighborhoods.

A series of national and regional learning convenings and site visits, along with virtual trainings and supports, forms the basis of the learning community.

Signs of progress in many *Invest Health* cities were evident after 12 months, with collaboration and action starting to take hold. Functional cross-sector partnerships in an increasing number of city teams were testing new ways of working together to plan, prioritize, and secure funding and financing for built environment projects.

A key theme emerging from the learning taking place through the ongoing developmental evaluation is that it takes time and patience to develop trust and build relationships across different sectors. While public officials, community developers, and others have been working in low-income neighborhoods for a long time, their efforts have typically been on separate tracks. After a year of learning side by side about the use of data to set common priorities, ways to impact the upstream factors of health through built environment projects, and strategies for accessing capital financing, the *Invest Health* cities are poised to advance investable opportunities through tangible projects. Two examples illustrate these efforts:

- **Akron, Ohio,** is a former manufacturing center that has been working to rebuild its economic strength. But the city's Middlebury neighborhood—where 40 percent of residents live in poverty and the average life expectancy is 10 years lower than the overall county average—has not been included in recent revitalization efforts.

  Akron's *Invest Health* team, which includes city government, local housing and community development organizations, and a local health system, is now prioritizing this community and working with it to identify strategies for rebuilding the central business district, increasing and improving housing options, and turning an abandoned railroad track into a hiking and biking path connected to adjacent neighborhoods.
- The **Richmond, Virginia,** *Invest Health* team is composed of a local health foundation, the public housing authority, two major health systems, and several city agencies. The collaboration started with a plan to redevelop a dilapidated public housing project into a walkable, mixed-income community with access to social services, green space, and a new grocery store. The team's experience with *Invest Health* then led it to embrace a larger goal of advancing a pipeline of projects across the city.

  These projects embed principles of health and equity with the dual goal of disrupting the concentrated pockets of poverty in its public housing developments and ensuring long-term housing affordability for current residents. *Invest Health* Richmond is also strategically using local housing market data to inform local housing policy and target limited capital to areas of need.

Cities like Akron, Richmond, and others with *Invest Health* teams are forging ahead into new territory to improve health and well-being in low-income neighborhoods. Their strategies are helping to illustrate what it means and takes to align community development, local government, health care, and public sector team members around a common vision for health and well-being and to pursue the type of sustainable systems and policy changes necessary to create more equitable communities.

The 18-month learning community ended in December 2017, but for many of these cities, this work is just a beginning. RWJF, in conjunction with the Reinvestment Fund, evaluation firm Mt. Auburn Associates, and the 50 participating cities, will be gathering and sharing the lessons from this initiative in 2018.

Working Together in a New Way With a Long-Term Partner

Building alliances across sectors requires creativity, patience, and the openness to venture outside one's comfort zone. RWJF and the YMCA of the USA (Y-USA) started working together more than nine years ago to help kids eat healthfully and move more. Through that work, both partners learned how to mobilize local YMCAs to inform policy, systems, and environmental change to support those goals.

As the vision for a Culture of Health crystalized, RWJF and Y-USA realized that they were undervaluing and underutilizing what their organizations could do together. Y-USA had a new CEO, and RWJF had begun to understand what it would take to shift from a national culture of illness-focused medical care to a Culture of Health. Both agreed it was time to think differently about how they worked together and move beyond their existing strategies.

In January 2015, Y-USA chief executive officer Kevin Washington and then RWJF president and chief executive officer Risa Lavizzo-Mourey, MD, MBA, charged staff with exploring opportunities to leverage the power, capacity, networks, and impact of the two organizations more fully. This was a new way of doing business for both—engaging staff across units (from program, communications, and research) to take the time to truly understand what they collectively bring to the table and what it would take to create a mutually beneficial partnership, not a traditional grantor–grantee relationship.

Both discovered ways they could work together that would strengthen their organizations and mobilize local YMCAs to strengthen local communities. These included better connecting YMCA health programs to health care providers and insurers and building on Y-USA's success with diabetes prevention; discovering new ways to nurture the potential of all children, parents, and caregivers, regardless of who they are or where they live, through Y-USA's early childhood programs; and elevating the importance of diversity, equity, and inclusion to community vibrancy and prosperity.

At the same time, both have been attentive to shaping conversations across the nation about health being more than what happens in the doctor's office by, for example, featuring Y-USA at the Aspen Ideas Festival and local YMCAs in Culture of Health Prize–winning communities. Together, both organizations have designed and launched a management services organization to pave the way for local YMCAs and other community-based organizations to transform access to preventive services.

RWJF and Y-USA fit as partners in a seamless and natural way, working toward the same end. Y-USA's mission clearly aligns with RWJF's vision. It reaches and activates various audiences to change communities, spread important principles and practices, and give the nation keen insights into what it takes to actually get that done. RWJF sees relationships like the one with Y-USA as essential to strengthen organizations that can mobilize action and build the momentum necessary to achieve a Culture of Health. Y-USA has taught RWJF what it means to work differently inside and outside of its walls.

At the same time, the RWJF team helps expand Y-USA's thinking and practices and provides a way for its teams to problem-solve. RWJF has been a catalyst for organizational change at Y-USA. Both partners believe that this increased effectiveness strengthens community—Y-USA's cause.

Positive, lasting, personal, and social change can only come about when everyone works together to invest in our kids, our health, and our neighbors. RWJF and Y-USA continue to find ways to advance one another's thinking and to be thought leaders about what it will take to strengthen America's communities as inclusive, healthy places to live, learn, work, and play.

Assessing the Uptake and Spread of the Culture of Health

RWJF is committed to understanding the extent to which the principles upon which the Culture of Health vision and Action Framework were developed—those around improving health and well-being and achieving health equity—are spreading throughout communities, organizations, and sectors across the nation, and to understanding how that diffusion is happening.

To help develop this understanding, RWJF commissioned George Grob, MA, president of the Center for Public Program Evaluation, to assess the early uptake of the Culture of Health vision, Action Framework, and principles of health equity.[3] Contracted evaluators gathered insights from diverse individuals and organizations working with RWJF that are likely to "both contribute to and be influenced by the Culture of Health." These included RWJF staff; partners, grantees, and former grantees; city mayors and health department officials; organizations in the health sector; and organizations in related non-health sectors.

The center's overall assessment is that "RWJF has made considerable progress" in its efforts to launch the Culture of Health vision and Action Framework. RWJF has changed the way it operates and garnered commitment among its own staff; it has continued to refine its messages and expand communications efforts to reach diverse audiences. "There are tentative but concrete signs that [the Culture of Health] is beginning to spread," the center reported to RWJF.

However, the widespread integration of the Culture of Health faces many challenges, including a complex and inequitable health care system and the charged sociopolitical climate.

Highlights of the evaluation:

- Familiarity with Culture of Health concepts is widespread among RWJF grantees, other organizations in the health sector, health-related organizations, and city health commissioners (from cities with populations greater than 50,000) who participated in the evaluation activities. Those who are familiar with the concepts strongly agree with them.
- City mayors and city health commissioners (from cities with populations greater than 50,000) who responded to the survey reported taking "deliberate action" in each of the four Action Areas of the Culture of Health Action Framework, rating their efforts at more than 3.5 on a 5-point scale.
- Although the concept of health equity is widely embraced and understood, city mayors and health commissioners (from cities with populations greater than 50,000) differ on the potential for policies at the city and county levels to impact health inequity in their communities, with 70 percent of mayors and 92 percent of health commissioners, among those who responded to the survey, agreeing that they can. Approximately 33 percent of mayors who responded defined equity as equal access to health care.

To build on the progress made thus far and to foster a broad social movement, the evaluation concluded, greater clarity on RWJF's efforts to build a Culture of Health and concrete examples, beyond grantmaking, of strategies and practices that effectively work to address the many complex determinants that impact health, well-being, and equity would be helpful to diverse stakeholders.

A Final Word

As a movement and a vision, the Culture of Health will require generations to achieve, but some progress on the journey to address health, well-being, and equity is evident—and there is much more yet to do.

Conclusion

ALONZO L. PLOUGH, PHD, MPH, MA
*Chief Science Officer and Vice President,
Research-Evaluation-Learning, Robert Wood Johnson Foundation*

As the Epilogue states, the Robert Wood Johnson Foundation embarked on a journey to build a Culture of Health in America in 2014. The inaugural *Sharing Knowledge to Build a Culture of Health* conference, held in Baltimore in March 2016, marked a key milestone along that journey, allowing us to engage with people we had not met before as well as with colleagues we have known for years. We continue to be enlightened and enriched by those associations and collaborations.

Much has changed since then. And, as this book goes to press, uncertainty prevails. The problems addressed throughout the book—lack of employment, inadequate health care, effects of climate change, incarceration, and others—do not adhere to political, geographic, or professional boundaries. They affect people who vote in red states and blue states, who live in rural villages and urban hubs, and who work in the professions or the trades.

The challenges in achieving health equity documented throughout the book reflect that too many communities experience feelings of despair. We are tempted to turn inward, feeling safe only when we engage with people whose views mirror our own. Heated disputes about the nature of "facts" leads to questioning, if not rejecting, the use of sound scientific evidence in making decisions.

Those observations, however, overlook the resiliency that is also a characteristic of this country. Through compelling presentations drawing on solid evidence and powerful personal narrative, contributors to this volume deliver a richer, more nuanced, and more hopeful perspective about the state of our union and our people. They remind us that ideas and passion continue to live and thrive in towns, suburbs, and urban centers across the country. They offer sound strategies for engaging in nontraditional collaborations that help us promote and sustain honest dialogue.

The stories you have read here testify to the reality of present-day turbulence, but they also offer a compass to help us navigate that turbulence through evidence and collective community action. They remind us that, despite our differences, Americans want everyone to be healthy and to thrive. Without underestimating the challenges that lie ahead, and aware that entrenched inequities have made our playing fields profoundly unfair, the contributors shine a light on meaningful accomplishments of inspired and inspiring citizens, policymakers, and researchers. They are stepping boldly into uncharted territory in order to generate and apply knowledge in the interest of equity and better lives for people.

We hope the book will serve as an inspiration and a resource manual on how improved health, well-being, and equity may be achieved.

ACKNOWLEDGMENTS

The *Sharing Knowledge to Build a Culture of Health* conference involved the hard work of numerous individuals, both internal and external to the Robert Wood Johnson Foundation. Priya Gandhi, MS, led the development of this conference, and Brian C. Quinn, PhD, provided leadership throughout the planning process. Lisa Simpson, MB, BCh, MPH, FAAP, and her staff at AcademyHealth collaborated with us to successfully convene this conference. I also want to thank the external steering committee who helped develop the sessions.

Turning the second annual conference into a book also required the vision and support of many. The Editorial Review Group oversees the development of this series and provided careful commentary and suggestions for this volume. My colleagues in this group are:

Sandro Galea, MD, MPH, DPH, Boston University
Sherry Glied, PhD, MA, New York University
Frederick Mann, Robert Wood Johnson Foundation
James Marks, MD, MPH, (formerly with) Robert Wood Johnson Foundation
Chad Zimmerman, Oxford University Press

Additional thanks to the team at the Robert Wood Johnson Foundation who provided leadership throughout the production of this manuscript:

Tanya Barrientos
Priya Gandhi, MS
Ed Ghisu, JD
Sofia Kounelias
Richard Besser, MD
Brian C. Quinn, PhD
Kristin Silvani

Finally, the following editorial consultants greatly supported the development of this manuscript:

Karyn Feiden
Mary B. Geisz, PhD
Karen Gross
Margaret O. Kirk
Mary Nakashian, MS

REFERENCES

Introduction

1. Pew Research Center. Public Trust in Government: 1958–2017. www.people-press.org/2017/05/03/public-trust-in-government-1958-2017/. Accessed October 23, 2017.

Section I

1. Pew Research Center. *More Americans Say Government Should Ensure Health Care Coverage* (2017). Washington: Pew Research Center. www.pewresearch.org/fact-tank/2017/01/13/more-americans-say-government-should-ensure-health-care-coverage/.
2. Pew Research Center. *Most Americans Say Economic System Unfairly Favors Powerful Interests* (2016). Washington: Pew Research Center. www.pewresearch.org/fact-tank/2016/02/10/most-americans-say-u-s-economic-system-is-unfair-but-high-income-republicans-disagree/ft_16-02-10_econsystem_party.
3. Pew Research Center. *Views About Whether Whites Benefit from Societal Advantages Split Sharply along Racial and Partisan Lines* (2017). Washington: Pew Research Center. www.pewresearch.org/fact-tank/2017/09/28/views-about-whether-whites-benefit-from-societal-advantages-split-sharply-along-racial-and-partisan-lines/.
4. Washington Post and Kaiser Family Foundation. *Survey of Rural America* (2017). Washington and Menlo Park, Calif: Washington Post and Kaiser Family Foundation. apps.washingtonpost.com/g/page/national/washington-post-kaiser-family-foundation-rural-and-small-town-america-poll/2217.
5. Kaiser Family Foundation and CNN. *Working Class Whites Poll* (2016). Menlo Park, Calif., and Washington: Kaiser Family Foundation and CNN. https://www.documentcloud.org/documents/3112930-8922-T-Kaiser-Family-Foundation-CNN-Working.html.

Chapter 1

1. Kneebone E, Holmes N. *US Concentrated Poverty in the Wake of the Great Recession* (2016). Washington: The Brookings Institution. https://www.brookings.edu/research/u-s-concentrated-poverty-in-the-wake-of-the-great-recession/.
2. Congressional Budget Office. *The Long-Term Budget Outlook* (2009). Washington: Congressional Budget Office. www.cbo.gov/sites/default/files/cbofiles/ftpdocs/102xx/doc10297/06-25-ltbo.pdf.
3. Mallaby S. "Progressive Wal-Mart. Really." *Washington Post.* November 28, 2005. www.washingtonpost.com/wp-dyn/content/article/2005/11/27/AR2005112700687.html.

Chapter 2

1. The Equality of Opportunity Project. Home page. www.equality-of-opportunity.org.
2. Chetty R, Hendren N, Kline P, Saez E. "Where Is the Land of Opportunity? The Geography of Intergenerational Mobility in the United States." *The Quarterly Journal of Economics.* 2014;129(4):1553–1623. https://doi.org/10.1093/qje/qju022.
3. Corak M, Heisz A. "The Intergenerational Earnings and Income Mobility of Canadian Men: Evidence from Longitudinal Income Tax Data." *Journal of Human Resources.* 1999:34(3):504–533.
4. Boserup SH, Kopczuk W, Kreiner CT. *Intergenerational Wealth Mobility: Evidence from Danish Wealth Records of Three Generations* (2013). Copenhagen: University of Copenhagen web.econ.ku.dk/eprn_epru/Seminar/WealthAcrossGen.pdf 2013.
5. Blanden J, Machin S. "Up and Down the Generational Income Ladder in Britain: Past Changes and Future Prospects." *National Institute Economic Review.* 2008:205(1):101–116. journals.sagepub.com/doi/10.1177/0027950108096594.
6. Chetty R, Hendren N. *The Impacts of Neighborhoods on Intergenerational Mobility I: Childhood Exposure Effects* (2016). National Bureau of Economic Research. www.equality-of-opportunity.org/assets/documents/movers_paper1.pdf.
7. Chetty R, Hendren N, Katz L. "The Effects of Exposure to Better Neighborhoods on Children: New Evidence from the Moving to Opportunity Experiment." *American Economic Review.* 2016;106(4):855–902. https://www.aeaweb.org/articles?id=10.1257/aer.20150572.
8. Chetty R, Stepner M, Abraham S, et al. "The Association Between Income and Life Expectancy in the United States, 2001–2014." *Journal of the American Medical Association.* 2016;315(16):1750–1766. jamanetwork.com/journals/jama/fullarticle/2513561?guestAccessKey=4023ce75-d0fb-44de-bb6c-8a10a30a6173.

Chapter 3

1. Mukai R, Lawrence S. *Foundation Funding for Native American Issues and Peoples* (2011). New York: Foundation Center. nativephilanthropy.org//wp-content/uploads/2013/03/2011-Foundation-Funding-for-Native-American-Issues-and-Peoples.pdf.
2. Stick C, Schaeffer M. *Native Strong. The Social Determinants of Health of Type 2 Diabetes and Obesity: A Research Framework* (2015). Santa Ana Pueblo, New Mexico: Notah Begay III Foundation. www.nb3foundation.org/assets/docs/2015-10-20-SDOH%20Full%20Summary%20FINAL.pdf.
3. Castellano M. "Updating Aboriginal Traditions of Knowledge." In Sefa Dei G, Hall B, Rosenberg D, eds. *Indigenous Knowledge in Global Contexts* (2000). Toronto: University of Toronto, 21–36.
4. Lloyd SA. "Court rules against Seattle's first-in-time law." *Curbed.* March 29, 2018. www.seattle.gov/Documents/Departments/CivilRights/socr-pr-060915.pdf
5. Martin JA, Hamilton BE, Osterman MJK. "Births in the United States, 2016." NCHS Data Brief. No, 287. September 2017. https://www.cdc.gov/nchs/data/databriefs/db287.pdf
6. Harrison MS, Goldenberg RL. "Global Burden of Prematurity." *Seminars on Fetal and Neonatal Medicine.* 2016 Apr;21(2):74–79. doi: 10.1016/j.siny.2015.12.007. Epub 2015 Dec 28. CC CERCCDOI: https://doi.org/10.1016/j.siny.2015.12.007.
7. Cunningham S, Lewis J, Thomas J, et al. "Expect With Me: Development and Evaluation Design for an Innovative Model of Group Prenatal Care to Improve Perinatal Outcomes." *BMC Pregnancy & Childbirth.* 2017;17(1):147. https://www.ncbi.nlm.nih.gov/pubmed/28521785.
8. Ickovics J, Kershaw T, Westdahl C, et al. "Group Prenatal Care and Perinatal Outcomes: A Randomized Controlled Trial." *Obstetrics & Gynecology.* 2007;110(4):330–339. journals.lww.com/greenjournal/Fulltext/2007/08000/Group_Prenatal_Care_and_Perinatal_Outcomes__A.17.aspx.
9. Kershaw TS, Magriples U, Westdahl C, Rising SS, Ickovics JR. "Pregnancy as a Window of Opportunity for HIV Prevention: Effects of an HIV Intervention Delivered Within Prenatal Care." *American Journal of Public Health.* 2009;99:2079–2086.

10. Ickovics J, Earnshaw V, Lewis J, et al. "Cluster Randomized Controlled Trial of Group Prenatal Care: Perinatal Outcomes Among Adolescents in New York City Health Centers." *American Journal of Public Health* 2016;106:359–365. ajph.aphapublications.org/doi/abs/10.2105/AJPH.2015.302960.

11. Magriples U, Boynton M, Kershaw T, et al. "The Impact of Group Prenatal Care on Pregnancy and Postpartum Weight Trajectories." *American Journal of Obstetrics and Gynecology.* 2015;213(5):688. https://www.ncbi.nlm.nih.gov/pubmed/26164694.

12. Felder J, Epel E, Lewis J, et al. "Depressive Symptoms and Gestational Length Among Pregnant Adolescents: Cluster Randomized Control Trial of CenteringPregnancy® Plus Group Prenatal Care." *Journal of Consulting and Clinical Psychology.* 2017;85(6):574–584. https://www.ncbi.nlm.nih.gov/pubmed/28287802.; Cole-Lewis H, Kershaw T, Earnshaw V, et al. "Pregnancy-Specific Stress, Preterm Birth, and Gestational Age Among High-Risk Young Women." *Health Psychology.* 2014;33(9):1033–1045. https://www.ncbi.nlm.nih.gov/pubmed/24447189.

13. Cunningham SD, Lewis JB, Shebl F, et al. "Impact of Group Prenatal Care on Preterm Birth and Low Birthweight: Propensity-Score Matched Study." [under review]

14. Carpenter Z. "What's Killing America's Black Infants?" *The Nation.* February 15, 2017. https://www.thenation.com/article/whats-killing-americas-black-infants/.

Chapter 4

1. Mays GP, Hoover AG, Ziliak JP, et al. *Research Agenda: Delivery and Financing System Innovations for a Culture of Health* (2015). Lexington, Ky.: Systems for Action National Program Office and Robert Wood Johnson Foundation. www.systemsforaction.org/projects/research-agenda/reports/systems-action-research-agenda.

2. Bloom D, Loprest PF, Zedlewski SR. *TANF Recipients with Barriers to Employment* (2011). Washington: Urban Institute.

3. Bloom SL. *Creating Sanctuary: Toward the Evolution of Sane Societies.*(2013). New York: Routledge.

4. Drexel University Center for Hunger-Free Communities. *The Building Wealth and Health Network: A Trauma-Informed Financial Self-Empowerment Program for Families with Young Children* (2016). Philadelphia: Drexel University Center for Hunger-Free Communities. http://www.centerforhungerfreecommunities.org/sites/default/files/pdfs/network_expanded_info_sheet1.pdf.

5. The Health Foundation. *Healthy Lives for People in the UK: Introducing the Health Foundation's Healthy Lives Strategy* (2017). London: The Health Foundation. http://www.health.org.uk/publication/healthy-lives-people-uk.

Chapter 5

1. The Sentencing Project, http://www.sentencingproject.org/issues/incarceration/.

2. http://www.sentencingproject.org/criminal-justice-facts/.

3. Harris C, Ortenburger M, Santiago F, et al. *Juvenile InJustice: Charging Youth as Adults Is Ineffective, Biased, and Harmful* (2017). Oakland, Calif.: Human Impact Partners. http://www.humanimpact.org/wp-content/uploads/HIP_JuvenileInJusticeReport_2017.02.pdf.

4. Mumola C, Karberg J. *Drug Use and Dependence, State and Federal Prisoners, 2004* (2007). Washington: U.S. Department of Justice. https://www.bjs.gov/content/pub/pdf/dudsfp04.pdf.

5. Karberg J, James D. *Substance Dependence, Abuse, and Treatment of Jail Inmates, 2002* (2005). Washington: U.S. Department of Justice. https://www.bjs.gov/content/pub/pdf/sdatji02.pdf.

6. Hughes T, Wilson D. *Reentry Trends in the United States: Inmates Returning to the Community after Serving Time in Prison* (2017). Washington: Bureau of Justice Statistics. https://www.bjs.gov/content/reentry/reentry.cfm.

7. National Institute of Justice. Recidivism. https://www.nij.gov/topics/corrections/recidivism/Pages/welcome.aspx. Accessed on December 18, 2017.

8. Wagner P. *Jails Matter. But Who Is Listening?* Northampton, Mass.: Prison Policy Initiative. Accessed on December 18, 2017. https://www.prisonpolicy.org/blog/2015/08/14/jailsmatter/.

9. Binswanger IA, et al. "Release from Prison: A High Risk of Death for Former Inmates." *New England Journal of Medicine.* 2007;356:157–165.

10. Wang EA, Hong CS, Shavit S, et al. "Engaging Individuals Recently Released from Prison Into Primary Care: A Randomized Trial." *American Journal of Public Health.* 2012;102(9):e22–e29.

11. Harris, et al., *Juvenile InJustice.*

12. National Criminal Justice Initiatives Map. https://csgjusticecenter.org/reentry/national-criminal-justice-initiatives-map/.

Chapter 6

1. Intergovernmental Panel on Climate Change. *Climate Change 2007: Synthesis Report* (Figures 2–3) (2007). Valencia, Spain: Intergovernmental Panel on Climate Change. https://www.ipcc.ch/pdf/assessment-report/ar4/syr/ar4_syr.pdf.

2. United States Environmental Protection Agency. "Sources of Greenhouse Gas Emissions" (2015). In: *Green House Gas Emissions.* Washington: United States Environmental Protection Agency. https://www.epa.gov/ghgemissions/sources-greenhouse-gas-emissions.

3. Maro P, Smith D, Acquarone A. *Acting Now for Better Health: A 30% Reduction Target for EU Climate Policy* (2010). Brussels, Belgium: The Health and Environmental Alliance and Health Care Without Harm, https://noharm.org/sites/default/files/lib/downloads/climate/Acting_Now_for_Better_Health.pdf.

Chapter 7

1. LaVeist TA, Gaskin DJ, Richard P. *The Economic Burden of Health Inequities in the United States* (2009). Washington: Joint Center for Political and Economic Studies. http://www.hhnmag.com/ext/resources/inc-hhn/pdfs/resources/Burden_Of_Health_FINAL_0.pdf.

2. Gaskin DJ, LaVeist TA, Richard P. *The State of Urban Health: Eliminating Health Disparities to Save Lives and Cut Costs* (2012). Washington: National Urban League Policy Institute. http://nulwb.iamempowered.com/sites/nulwb.iamempowered.com/files/NUL%20SOUH%20Final%20%282012%29.pdf.

3. Turner A. *The Business Case for Racial Equity in Michigan* (2015). Battle Creek, Mich.: W. K. Kellogg Foundation. http://altarum.org/sites/default/files/uploaded-publication-files/Business%20Case%20for%20Racial%20Equity%20in%20Michigan_May%202015.pdf.

4. Turner A, LaVeist T, Gaskin D, et al. *Economic Impacts of Health Disparities in Texas* (2016). Houston: Episcopal Health Foundation and San Antonio: Methodist Healthcare Ministries of South Texas Inc. http://www.episcopalhealth.org/files/7314/8106/4634/Economic_Impact_Report_EHF_and_MHM_Logos_FINAL.pdf.

5. NEJM Catalyst. http://catalyst.nejm.org/predictive-analytics-determine-next-years-highest-cost-patients/. Accessed October 23, 2017.

6. NEJM Catalyst. http://catalyst.nejm.org/health-care-that-targets-unmet-social-needs/. Accessed October 23, 2017.

7. NEJM Catalyst (catalyst.nejm.org). Copyright Massachusetts Medical Society. Data reflect response rates as of March 4, 2016.

8. Moneyball for Government: The Book. http://moneyballforgov.com/moneyball-for-government-the-book/. Accessed October 23, 2017.

Chapter 8

1. U.S. Atlas on General Election Turnout (2012). https://uselectionatlas.org/RESULTS/national.php?year=2012

2. U.S. Current Population Survey (2013). https://www.nationalservice.gov/about/open-government-initiative/open-government-gallery.

3. U.S. Current Population Survey (2013). https://www.nationalservice.gov/about/open-government-initiative/open-government-gallery.

4. Bye L, Ghirardelli A. *American Health Values Survey* (2016). Princeton, N.J.: Robert Wood Johnson Foundation. http://www.rwjf.org/en/library/research/2016/06/american-health-values-survey-topline-report.html.

5. Plough AL (ed.). *Knowledge to Action: Accelerating Progress in Health, Well-Being, and Equity* (2017). New York: Oxford University Press.

6. Commission on Social Determinants of Health. *Closing the Gap in a Generation* (2008). Geneva: World Health Organization. http://www.who.int/social_determinants/thecommission/finalreport/en/.

Chapter 10

1. Higashi RT, Craddock Lee SJ, Leonard T, et al. "Multiple Comorbidities and Interest in Research Participation among Clients of a Nonprofit Food Distribution Site." *Clinical and Translational Science.* 2015;8(5):584–590. http://dx.doi.org/10.1111/cts.12325. Higashi RT, Craddock Lee SJ, Pezzia C, et al. "Family and Social Context Contributes to the Interplay of Economic Insecurity, Food Insecurity, and Health." *Annals of Anthropology Practice.* (In press.)

2. Scally CP, Waxman E, Gourevitch R, et al. *Emerging Strategies for Integrating Health and Housing: Innovations to Sustain, Expand, and Replicate* (2017). Washington: Urban Institute.

3. Scally CP, Waxman E, Gourevitch R. *Good Neighbors Make Better Partners: Columbus, Ohio* (2017). Washington: Urban Institute.

4. Scally CP, Waxman E, Adeeyo S. *Everything in One Place: Washington, DC* (2017). Washington: Urban Institute.

5. Scally CP, Waxman E, Gourevitch R. *A City Takes Action: Boston, Massachusetts* (2017). Washington: Urban Institute.

6. Scally CP, Waxman E, Gourevitch R. *A National Insurer Goes Local* (2017). Washington: Urban Institute.

Chapter 11

1. Friedman D, Perry D, Menendez C. *The Foundational Role of Universities as Anchor Institutions in Urban Development—A Report of National Data and Survey Findings* (2014). Washington: The Coalition of Urban Serving Universities and the Association of Public and Land-Grant Universities. http://usucoalition.org/images/APLU_USU_Foundational_FNLlo.pdf.

2. Tavernise S. "Disparity in Life Spans of the Rich and the Poor Is Growing." *New York Times.* February 12, 2016. www.nytimes.com/2016/02/13/health/disparity-in-life-spans-of-the-rich-and-the-poor-is-growing.html.

3. Kochhar R, Fry R. *Wealth Inequality Has Widened Along Racial, Ethnic Lines since End of Great Recession* (2014). Washington: Pew Research Center. www.pewresearch.org/fact-tank/2014/12/12/racial-wealth-gaps-great-recession.

4. Glanville J. *Cleveland's Greater University Circle Initiative: A Partnership Between Philanthropy, Anchor Institutions, and the Public Sector* (2014). Cleveland: The Cleveland Foundation.

5. Zuckerman D, et al. *Hospitals Building Healthier Communities—Embracing the Anchor Mission* (2013). Washington: Democracy Collaborative. http://democracycollaborative.org/content/hospitals-building-healthier-communities-embracing-anchor-mission.

6. Harkavy I, Zuckerman H. *Eds and Meds: Cities' Hidden Assets* (1999). Washington: The Brookings Institution Center on Urban and Metropolitan Policy. http://community-wealth.org/search-ex/Eds%20and%20Meds%3A%20Cities%27%20Hidden%20Assets.

7. Zuckerman, et al. *Hospitals Building Healthier Communities.*

8. Friedman, et al. *Foundational Role of University as Anchor Institutions in Urban Development.*

Chapter 12

1. Mariner W, Annas GJ. "A Culture of Health and Human Rights." *Health Affairs.* 2016;35:1999–2004. http://content.healthaffairs.org/content/35/11/1999.abstract.
2. Huang T, Sorenson D, Davis S, et al. "Healthy Eating Design Guidelines for School Architecture." *Preventing Chronic Disease.* 2013;10:120084. https://www.cdc.gov/pcd/issues/2013/pdf/12_0084.pdf.
3. Brittin J, Sorenson D, Trowbridge M, et al. "Physical Activity Design Guidelines for School Architects." *PLOS One.* 2015;10(7):e132597. http://journals.plos.org/plosone/article?id=10.1371/journal.pone.0132597.
4. Trowbridge M, Worden K, Pyke C. "Using Green Building as a Model for Making Health Promotion Standard in the Built Environment." *Health Affairs.* 2016;35(11):2062–2067. http://content.healthaffairs.org/content/35/11/2062.abstract.

Chapter 13

1. Wilsdon J, Bar-Ilan J, Frodeman R, et al. *Next-Generation Metrics: Responsible Metrics and Evaluation for Open Science* (2017). Luxembourg: Publications Office of the European Union. https://ec.europa.eu/research/openscience/pdf/report.pdf.

Section V

1. 2017 County Health Rankings: Kentucky. http://www.countyhealthrankings.org/sites/default/files/state/downloads/CHR2017_KY.pdf. Accessed October 23, 2017.
2. Sommeiller E, Price M, Wazeter E. *Income Inequality in the US by State, Metropolitan Area, and County* (2016). Washington: Economic Policy Institute. http://www.epi.org/publication/income-inequality-in-the-us/.

Chapter 15

1. *Health in Louisville Metro Neighborhoods* (2014). Louisville, Ky.: Center for Health Equity. https://louisvilleky.gov/sites/default/files/health_and_wellness/che/health_equity_report/her2014_7_31_14.pdf.
2. Plough A. *Clearing the Air in Louisville Through Data and Design* (2015). Princeton, N.J.: Robert Wood Johnson Foundation. https://www.rwjf.org/en/culture-of-health/2015/05/clearing_the_airin.html.
3. Network Center for Community Change. West Louisville Neighborhood Data. http://makechangetogether.org/data/. Accessed December 18, 2017.
4. Arno C, Rock P. *Louisville Metro Health Equity Report: The Social Determinants of Health in Louisville Metro Neighborhoods.*
5. Poe J. Redlining Louisville: The History of Race, Class, and Real Estate. https://lojic.maps.arcgis.com/apps/MapSeries/index.html?appid=e4d29907953c4094a17cb9ea8f8f89de. Accessed December 15, 2017.
6. 55,000 Degrees. http://www.55000degrees.org/about-55k/faqs/. Accessed December 18, 2017.
7. Humana. http://populationhealth.humana.com/louisville/, from the Louisville Health Advisory Board. Accessed December 18, 2017.
8. Slabaugh S, Shah M, Zack M, et al. "Leveraging Health-Related Quality of Life in Population Health Management: The Case for Healthy Days." *Population Health Management.* 2017;20(1):13–22. https://www.medscape.com/medline/abstract/27031869.

Chapter 16

1. Lowrey A. "What's the Matter With Eastern Kentucky?" *New York Times Magazine*, June 26, 2014. https://www.nytimes.com/2014/06/29/magazine/whats-the-matter-with-eastern-kentucky.html?mcubz=1&_r=0.
2. Kentucky Rankings data. http://www.countyhealthrankings.org/rankings/data/ky.
3. Culhane D, Metraux S, Hadley T. *Public Service Reductions Associated with Placement of Homeless Persons with Severe Mental Illness in Supportive Housing* (2002). Philadelphia: Fannie Mae Foundation. https://shnny.org/uploads/The_Culhane_Report.pdf.

Epilogue

1. Besser, Richard. 2017. "New Leadership at the Robert Wood Johnson Foundation." Speech given at the Aspen Ideas Festival, Aspen, Colo., Friday, June 23, 2017. https://www.aspenideas.org/sites/default/files/transcripts/New%20Leadership%20at%20the%20Robert%20Wood%20Johnson%20Foundation_0.pdf.
2. Plough A, Miller C, Tait M. *Moving Forward Together* (2018). Princeton, N.J.: Robert Wood Johnson Foundation.
3. Grob G. *Building a Culture of Health Progress Report, Year One* (2018). Princeton, N.J.: Robert Wood Johnson Foundation.

INDEX